医护人员诊疗英语会话

Conversational English for the Hospital

主　编　李　婷　李　娜

副主编　陆　垚　谈晓轶　张之薇

（以下按姓氏笔画顺序）

编　者　于银磊　刘　坤　李　青

　　　　陆丽英　肖　凡　张　蓓

　　　　周思源　贾留全　甄晓婕

 南京大学出版社

图书在版编目(CIP)数据

医护人员诊疗英语会话 / 李婷,李娜主编. — 南京:
南京大学出版社,2020.7
　　ISBN 978-7-305-23378-4

　　Ⅰ. ①医… Ⅱ. ①李… ②李… Ⅲ. ①医学－英语－
口语－自学参考资料 Ⅳ. ①R

中国版本图书馆 CIP 数据核字(2020)第 092202 号

出版发行	南京大学出版社
社　　址	南京市汉口路 22 号　　　　邮　编　210093
出 版 人	金鑫荣
书　　名	**医护人员诊疗英语会话**
主　　编	李婷 李娜
责任编辑	裴维维　　　　　　编辑热线　025-83592123
照　　排	南京南琳图文制作有限公司
印　　刷	常州市武进第三印刷有限公司
开　　本	787×960　1/16　印张 11　字数 230 千
版　　次	2020 年 7 月第 1 版　2020 年 7 月第 1 次印刷

ISBN 978-7-305-23378-4
定　　价　39.80 元

网址:http://www.njupco.com
官方微博:http://weibo.com/njupco
官方微信号:njupress
销售咨询热线:(025)83594756

总　序

　　在中华民族迎来伟大复兴的光明前景下，建设教育强国是这一时期一项重要的基础工程。围绕教育要"培养什么人、怎样培养人、为谁培养人"这个根本问题，以及国务院办公厅《关于深化医教协同进一步推进医学教育改革和发展的意见》中关于强化医德素养和人文素质教育、整体提升医学教育办学能力和人才培养质量的相关要求，医学院校的学科体系、教学体系、教材体系、管理体系均需要围绕相关目标来设计。

　　英语教育作为高等教育的一个重要环节，在人才培养方面发挥着不可替代的作用，必须保持与时俱进、开拓创新，以满足学生专业学习、国际交流、继续深造、工作就业等方面的需求，这关系到高等教育人才培养的质量。相关课程设置不仅要满足专业需求，还需要符合国家大政方针，帮助学生树立世界眼光、培养国际意识，使之成为有理想、有本领、有担当的高素质专门人才，为实现中华民族伟大复兴的中国梦提供强有力的人才保障。对医学生而言，英语学习更是个系统工程，医学院校的大学本科和研究生英语都要落实"立德树人"这一根本任务，在教学理念、课程设置、教学模式等方面适应新时代英语教育教学的相关要求。

　　一、本系列教材体现现阶段高等教育人才培养需求。大学英语课程，尤其是医学院校大学英语课程，应该兼具工具性和人文性双重性质，应该具备满足学生跨文化交流的需要，以及学生在学术或者职业领域进行交流的需要。故本系列教材按照医学生在校学习及职业成长的主线，以相关语言技能的培养为轴,结合医学生的专业个性需求,分阶段、分模块、分层次展开设置,尽量满足不同层次医学生的学习需求。

二、本系列教材所选主题,注重语言文化教育与思政教育的结合,坚持价值性和知识性的统一、建设性和批判性的统一。除医学相关的基础内容外,本系列教材注重学生家国情怀、人文情怀的培养,注重医德与人文素质的培养,注重学生对问题的判断能力、分析能力和说服能力的培养。

三、本系列教材注重将语言学习还教于生,设计了多样的教学任务、教学活动与教学环节,借助现代信息技术,积极创建多元的教学与学习环境,利用当前已设置的微课、慕课等优质教学资源拓展教学内容,实施基于课堂和在线网上课程的翻转课堂等混合式教学模式,充分调动学生积极性。通过建立的网上交互学习平台,为师生提供涵盖课堂互动、教师辅导、学生练习、作业反馈、学习评估等环节的教学体系。

四、本系列教材除满足学生学习需求外,还设置了相应模块,满足学术交流、测评体系的需求,将相关主流考试的题型作为参考,体现在教材设置中。

本书编写组

前　言

　　近年来，随着全球化进程的加快和医学国际交流的不断深入，医务人员英语交流水平愈显重要。在工作中能顺利地用英语与外籍病人交谈以及开展问诊、检查、交代病情等诊疗活动，提高涉外医疗服务水平，是许多医务人员的迫切需求。本书面向国内广大医务人员，通过有针对性的学习训练，提高医学英语口语表达能力，强化医学英语环境下的沟通能力、社交能力及应变能力，使其能够更好地参与国际交流。

　　本书共分十个单元。一至三单元主要围绕医疗服务主题，四至十单元则以临床诊疗过程为依托，按诊疗顺序，即问诊、检查化验及诊断治疗几个步骤展开。每个单元都包含基本词汇与表达、对话模板、练习、其他有用句型、补充阅读及英语会话功能句型六个部分。附录部分则提供了医学英语口语中可能涉及的常用专业词汇。

　　本书总结出医学英语会话中各类具有代表性的基本句型，并通过形式多样的练习及丰富的词汇、句型、文章等素材进行学习强化，使学习者可以以此为依据，举一反三地应用于医院背景下各类医学英语会话之中。本书可作为医学院校英语口语教材或在职医务人员英语口语研修班教材，亦可作为医务人员的自学用书。

Contents
目 录

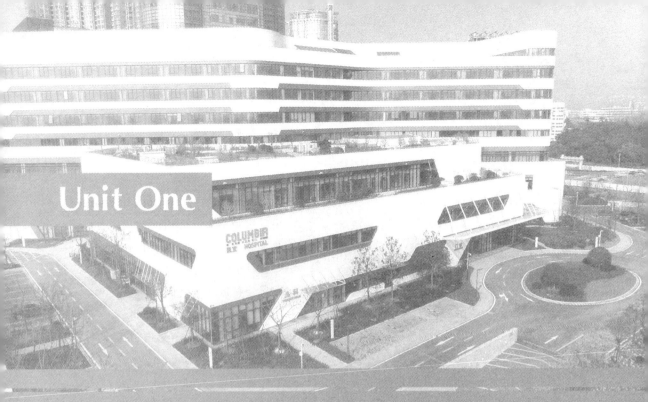

Unit One

Introducing Yourself as a Doctor
自我介绍

Learning Objectives

熟悉各科医生的英文说法

掌握与医生自我介绍相关的句型结构

了解医生自我介绍的正确方式及注意事项

Outline

✓音、视频资源

✓参考答案

✓学术探讨

Part One

Words and Expressions

内科医生	physician	主管医师	physician in charge
外科医生	surgeon	实习医师	intern
呼吸科医生	respiratory/ pulmonary physician	耳鼻喉科医生	ENT surgeon
		心脏科医生	cardiologist
血液科医生	hematologist	血管外科医生	vascular surgeon
肝脏科医生	hepatologist	儿科医生	pediatrician
泌尿科医生	urologist	妇科医生	gynecologist
产科医生	obstetrician	肿瘤科医生	oncologist
眼科医生	ophthalmologist	牙科医生	dentist
骨科医生	orthopedist	整形外科医生	plastic surgeon
皮肤科医生	dermatologist	神经科医生	neurologist
精神病医生	psychiatrist	病理科医生	pathologist
心理医生	psychologist	放射科医生	radiologist
麻醉科医生	anesthetist	技术人员	technician
药剂师	pharmacist	医护人员	medical staff
（科）主任	director/ head of the （department）	主任医师	chief physician
		主治医师	attending physician
副主任医师	associate chief physician	住院医师	resident

Part Two

Model Dialogues

Self-introduction 自我介绍

1. Hello! My name is Su Yin, and my English name is Mary. So you can call me Mary. I am a doctor of internal medicine. What can I do for you?

你好！我是苏医生，我的英文名叫玛丽。你可以叫我玛丽。我是内科医生，我能帮您做些什么？

2. Good Afternoon! My name is Dr. Wu. **I am a cardiac surgeon**，and **I am responsible for your treatment.**

下午好！我是吴医生。我是胸外科医生，我负责你的治疗。

3. Hi，**I am Dr. Tang**，and my English name is Grant. **Please call me Dr. Grant. I work in Gynecology Department**，and **I will be looking after you. May I help you**?

你好，我是唐医生。我的英文名叫格兰特，你可以叫我格兰特医生。我是一名妇科医生，将由我来负责你的诊疗。我可以帮你吗？

Useful Structures

1. My English name is Mary，so you can/please call me Mary.
   我的英文名叫玛丽，你可以/请称呼我玛丽。

2. I am Dr. Tang. I am a doctor of internal medicine.
   我是唐医生，我是内科的医生。

3. I am a cardiac surgeon.
   我是胸外科医生。

4. I work in Gynecology Department.
   我在妇科工作。

5. I am responsible for your treatment.
   我负责您疾病的治疗。

6. I will be looking after you.
   将由我来负责你的诊疗。

7. What can I do for you?
   我能帮您做些什么吗？

8. May I help you?
   我可以帮你吗？

Part Three
Exercises

• Put the following sentences or expressions into English.

1. 外科医生 _____ 2. 血液科医生 _____

3. 眼科医生 _____ 4. 骨科医生 _____

5. 神经科医生 _____ 6. 呼吸科医生 _____

7. 心脏科医生 _____ 8. 肿瘤科医生 _____

9. 皮肤科医生 _____ 10. 药剂师 _____

11. 我是一名儿科医生，我的病人都是儿童。

　　_____

12. 我是耳鼻喉科医生。ENT 代表的是耳鼻喉。

　　_____

13. 我是泌尿科医生凯特，我负责你的治疗。

　　_____

14. 她叫王梦，是我们的护士长。

　　_____

15. 这个部门的医生也叫作外科医生，他们给病人做手术。

　　_____

16. 内科医生主要用药物治疗病人。

　　_____

17. 医生是医院医疗的核心力量。

　　_____

18. 没有护士和技术人员的辅助，医生不可能给病人提供有效的医疗。

　　_____

• Fill in the blanks to complete the sentences.

1. Good morning, my name is Anna.

　　Please _____ me _____.

I _____ in the Internal Medicine Department.

Can I _____ you?

2. Good afternoon. My name is Dr. Wu.

I am a cardiac _____.

I am _____ for your _____.

Can you _____ me what your _____ is?

Part Four

Other Structures

1. Mr. Smith，I'd like you to meet ...

   史密斯先生，我想给你介绍······

2. Mr. Brown，may I introduce you to ...?

   布朗先生，我能为你介绍······吗?

3. Dr. Wang，I'd like to introduce ...

   王医生，我想介绍······

4. Miss White，can I introduce ...? He's the dean of the Foreign Language Department.

   怀特小姐，我来介绍······，他是外语学院的主任。

5. Dad，have you met Yang Ling? She's my classmate.

   爸爸，你见过杨玲吗? 她是我的同学。

6. Linda，meet Alex.

   琳达，这是艾利克斯。

7. Allow me to introduce myself. My name is ...

   请允许我介绍我自己，我的名字叫······

8. May I introduce myself? I'm Tom.

   我能介绍下我自己吗? 我叫汤姆。

Part Five

Supplementary Reading: The Right and Wrong Way to Introduce Yourself to Patients

When you meet a new patient, you'll need to introduce yourself. But for many nurses or doctors, this is easier said than done. If you're not exactly a social butterfly, meeting new people can be challenging. But the way you introduce yourself is important for patient relations, and you need to make a good impression to help the patient feel comfortable and at ease.

Your introduction forms the basis of your patient-provider relationship. Not only are your words and tone of voice important, but your body language also plays an important role. It's estimated in the textbook *Communication and Nursing* that about 85% of communication is primarily nonverbal. A lack of communication comes across as unprofessional, and it can make the patient feel uncomfortable. Being friendly, upbeat, and empathetic is essential when interacting with patients.

What's the Best Way to Introduce Yourself?

A great introduction can be described by the "five P's":

- You need to know who the patient is.
- Understand where people fall in a hierarchy, and how it's appropriate to address them.
- Develop a consistent introduction to use.
- Be sure to say the patient's name clearly and correctly.
- Introducing a point of commonality can go a long way toward forging a good connection with someone.

Here are some tips for a great personal introduction.

- Make eye contact and shake their hands. Making eye contact and shaking their hands helps you come across as friendly and personable.
- *Address them by an honorific*. Address your patients as "Mr." "Mrs." "Miss" and other honorifics, unless they specifically ask you to address them by their first name.

- *Make sure nonverbal communication is positive.* Your facial expressions, body posture, and degree of eye contact send out social signals. Sit or stand in a position where you're close to being eye to eye with patients. Lean slightly toward them, and avoid crossing your arms or legs.
- *Use the right tone of voice.* Make sure your tone comes across as interested, polite, and empathetic. Speak clearly, at a pace that is neither too fast nor too slow, and avoid using too much jargon.
- *Explain why you're there.* It's helpful for the patients to understand why you're seeing them. For example, "I've come to measure your blood pressure today." If you're performing any type of procedure, make sure the patient fully understands what you're doing, and that he/she consents to it.
- *Ask the patients if they have any questions.* Patients are sometimes hesitant to actively ask questions or bring up their concerns. Inviting them to do so can encourage them to open up, which may provide you with medically relevant information.
- *Ask if they need anything else.* Before you leave, ask the patients if there's anything else they need from you. Again, they may be hesitant to bring it up on their own.
- *Thank them, and explain what will happen next.* Saying "thank you" is only polite. You should also explain what's going to happen next — for example, whether the doctor will see them momentarily, or if you're going to come back again later.

How Not to Introduce Yourself

We've discussed the best ways to introduce yourself to a patient, but many nurses or doctors make mistakes that can damage their therapeutic relationship with their patients. Here are some of the most common introduction missteps.

- Not introducing yourself by name. It's surprising how often doctors and nurses neglect to give a patient their name. When you fail to introduce yourself, the patient may feel alienated.
- Coming across as cold and aloof. A warm, welcoming demeanor is a big part of good bedside manner. If you come across as uninterested or annoyed, it

makes patients uncomfortable.

- Ignoring patients or not listening to them. It's important to be a good listener. Some patients may seem to go on and on about things that don't matter, but it's polite to listen and nod your head anyway. Patients also voice concerns about things like pain or discomfort. It's important not to write off these complaints.

- Not explaining what you're doing. Patients can benefit from understanding what you're doing when you visit them. Whether you're administering a medication or examining their vital signs, it's alienating and uncomfortable when they aren't told what's going on.

A Great Introduction Can Make a Patient's Day

When you introduce yourself to patients, a warm greeting, and friendly demeanor can make a big difference for them. Whether they're in a hospital bed or they're seeing their GP for an annual check-up, patients can benefit when staff members are friendly and responsive.

Part Six

Conversational English Functions

- Greeting and Introducing 问候和介绍

1. Greeting

Hello!

Good morning/afternoon/evening.

How do you do?

Glad/Pleased/Delighted to meet you.

How are you?

How are things?

How have you been getting on?

How's it going?

How are you doing/keeping?

What's new?

What's up?

2. Introducing

Mr. Brown, I'd like you to meet ...

Mrs. White, may I introduce you to ... ?

Dr. Wang, I'd like to introduce ...

Miss Morgan, can I introduce ... ? He's the ...

Dad, have you met Yang Ling? She's ...

Linda, meet Alex.

Allow me to introduce myself. My name is ...

Hello, I'm ... from ...

May I introduce myself? I'm Tom.

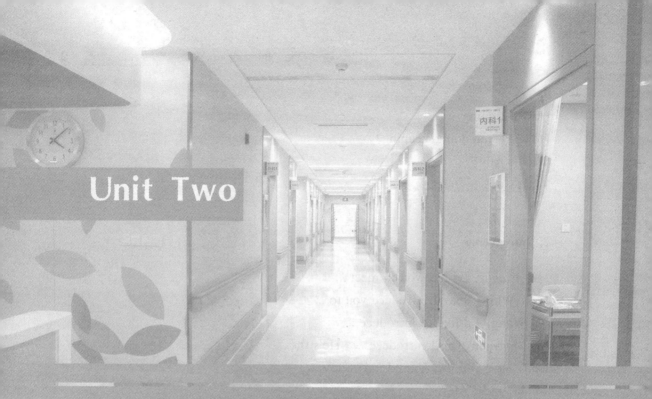

Unit Two

Departments and Directions
科室及问路

Learning Objectives

熟悉医院各科室英文名称

掌握医院情境下与问路相关的句型结构

了解不同文化背景下的问候方式

Outline

✓音、视频资源

✓参考答案

✓学术探讨

Part One

Words and Expressions

挂号	registration		(Department)
科室	department	检验科	Clinical Laboratory
急诊部	Emergency(Department)	心电图室	Electrocardiograph
门诊手术室	Operation Room of		(ECG) Room
	Outpatient Department	ECT 检查	ECT Scan
外科	Surgery (Department)	药房	Pharmacy
呼吸科	Respiratory Medicine	细菌室	Bacteriology
	(Department)	门诊部	Outpatient
放射科	Radiology (Department)		Department/
口腔科	Stomatology		Outpatients
	(Department)	住院部	Inpatient
眼科	Ophthalmology		Department
	(Department)	内科	Internal Medicine
耳鼻喉科	Ear，Nose & Throat/		(Department)
	E. N. T. (Department)	心脏科	Cardiology
产科	Obstetrics(Department)		(Department)
妇产科	Obstetric-gynecology	精神科	Psychiatry
	(Department)		(Department)
肿瘤科	Oncology	风湿科	Rheumatology
	(Department)		(Department)
泌尿科	Urology	神经科	Neurology
	(Department)		(Department)
血管外科	Vascular Surgery	皮肤科	Dermatology
	(Department)		(Department)
核医学科	Nuclear Medicine	内分泌科	Endocrinology
	(Department)		(Department)
理疗科	Physiotherapy	妇科	Gynecology

	(Department)			(Department)
儿科	Pediatrics		整形外科	Plastic Surgery
	(Department)			(Department)
消化内科	Gastroenterology/ Gastrology		病理科	Pathology
			换药室	Dressing Room
	(Department)		CT 室	CT Scan Room
血液科	Hematology		磁共振成像室	MRI Scan Room
	(Department)		超声科	Ultrasound
麻醉科	Anesthesiology			

Part Two

Model Dialogues

Dialogue One

Doctor：Hello! I am Dr. Lin. Can I help you?

医生：你好，我是林医生。我可以帮助你吗？

Patient：I want to see a doctor, please. I don't feel very well, but I don't know what to do.

病人：我需要看医生。我感觉不舒服,不知道该怎么办。

Doctor：What are your symptoms?

医生：你有哪些症状呢?

Patient：I have a temperature, and I am feeling tired and aching.

病人：我发烧,感觉酸痛乏力。

Doctor：**You need to see a doctor of Internal Medicine.** Do you understand Chinese?

医生：你需要看内科医生。你会讲中文吗?

Patient：No, I'm afraid not.

病人：不会。

Doctor：**You have to register first.** Then **I will take you to the Outpatient Department.**

医生：你需要先挂号，然后我带你去门诊部。

Patient：**Where is the registration office**?

病人：请问挂号处在哪?

Doctor：Go straight ahead，and you will see the registration office in front of you. **By the way，do you have a patient ID card**?

医生：一直走，挂号处就在你前面。顺便问一下，你有就诊卡吗?

Patient：No, I don't have one. This is my first time to this hospital.

病人：没有，这是我第一次来这个医院。

Doctor：**Then you need to go to the reception and fill in your personal information to get a medical card.**

医生：那你需要先去服务台填写个人信息办理就诊卡。

Patient：OK. Thank you very much.

病人：好的，非常感谢。

Dialogue Two

Doctor：Hello，may I help you? I am Dr. Lee.

医生：你好，我能帮助你吗? 我是李医生。

Patient：Yes，please! I have a severe headache. I need to see a doctor. Where do I have to go?

病人：是的，我头疼，需要看医生。我该去哪个科呢?

Doctor：You need to see a Neurologist，and **the Neurology Department is on the 4th floor.**

医生：你需要看神经科医生，神经科在四楼。

Patient：OK. Thank you. **Can you tell me where the elevator is，please**?

病人：好的，谢谢。你能告诉我电梯在哪里吗?

Doctor：**The elevators are over there around the corner. You just go down the corridor and then turn left. You will see them right in front of you.**

医生：电梯就在那边拐角处。你沿着走廊一直走然后左转，就能看到电梯在你面前。

Patient：Thank you so much.

病人：非常感谢。

Doctor：But you need to register first.

医生：但你需要先挂号。

Patient：Thank you. You are very kind, Dr. Lee.

病人：谢谢。你人真好,李医生。

Doctor：It's my pleasure.

医生：不客气。

Dialogue Three

Patient：Hello! I often feel a headache from time to time. **What department should I go**?

病人：您好,我常常感到头疼,应该挂什么科呢?

Nurse：Hello! **I suggest you register at the Neurology Department. Is this your first visit to our hospital**?

护士：您好! 建议您挂神经科,这是您第一次来我院就诊吗?

Patient：Yes. How can I get registered?

病人：是的,请问怎么挂号?

Nurse：If you have brought your ID card or any other valid documents, you can go to the registration windows directly. If not, **please fill in the Registration Form for the First Visit Patients**, and then confirm your identity at the verification desk on the right. Finally, **you can register at the registration windows.**

护士：如果您带了身份证或其他有效证件,可以直接到挂号窗口挂号,未带的话请填写好《初诊病人登记表》,然后到右边实名认证审核处核实身份后再去挂号。

Patient：OK. I would like to register with Dr. Liu, but he is not available now. What should I do?

病人：好的。我想挂刘主任的号,可是他的号已经挂不到了,我该怎么办?

Nurse：If you insist on Dr. Liu, there are two options. **You can go to his office to ask whether he could offer an extra registration** and then register at the window. He is now in Room 212 on the 2nd floor. Or you can make an appointment with him today for the next week.

护士：您一定要看刘主任门诊的话,有两个方法。一是您去他的诊间,请他帮您加号,然后再去挂号窗口挂号,他现在在 2 楼的 212 号房间;二是您今天可以挂他下周的预约号。

Patient：OK. Then how could I make a registration for the next week please?

病人：好的,请问我如何挂下周的号呢?

Nurse：You can either go to the registration window directly or just make a call or send messages with your mobile phone. Besides, **you may also register on the Internet or App**. You can come to the hospital on the appointed day, get a number and pay at the hospital after getting your appointed registration.

护士：您可以直接到挂号窗口挂号,也可以在家里通过电话、短信、网络、APP 等任意一种方式挂号,预约后你来医院取号缴费即可。

Patient：Thank you.

病人：谢谢。

Useful Structures

1. You need to see a doctor of Internal Medicine.
   你需要看内科医生。
2. You have to register first.
   你需要先挂号。
3. I will take you to the(Outpatient) Department.
   我带你去(门诊)部。
4. Where is the registration office?
   请问挂号处在哪?
5. Go straight ahead, and you will see the registration office in front of you.
   直走,挂号处就在你前面。
6. Then you need to go to the reception and fill in your personal information to get a medical card.
   那你需要先去服务台填写个人信息办理就诊卡。
7. The Neurology Department is on the 4th floor.
   神经科在四楼。

8. Can you tell me where the elevator is, please?

   你能告诉我电梯在哪吗?

9. The elevators are over there around the corner.

   电梯就在那边拐角处。

10. You just go down the corridor and then turn left.

    你沿着走廊一直走然后左转。

11. You will see the elevators right in front of you.

    你会看到电梯在你面前。

12. What department should I go?

    我应该挂什么科呢?

13. I suggest you register at the Neurology Department.

    我建议您挂神经科。

14. Is this your first visit to our hospital?

    这是您第一次来我院就诊吗?

15. Please fill in the Registration Form for the First Visit Patients.

    请填写《初诊病人登记表》。

16. You can register at the registration windows.

    你可以到挂号窗口挂号。

17. You can go to his office to ask whether he could offer an extra registration.

    您去他的诊间,请他帮您加号。

18. You may also register on the Internet or App.

    您可以在家里通过网络或APP方式挂号。

Part Three

Exercises

• Put the following sentences or expressions into English.

1. 精神科 _____   2. 风湿科 _____

3. 内分泌科 _____   4. 消化内科 _____

5. 麻醉科　_____　　6. 急诊室　_____

7. 心电图室　_____　　8. 放射科　_____

9. 口腔科　_____　　10. 儿科　_____

11. 泌尿科　_____　　12. 病理科　_____

13. 检验科　_____　　14. 磁共振成像室　_____

15. 你好,请问住院部在哪里?

_____

16. 我在找自动取款机,请问医院里面有吗?

_____

17. 心电图检查室在二楼。

_____

18. 沿着走廊一直走,就在你的右手边。

_____

19. 你可以坐电梯上去。

_____

20. 你需要先挂号,往前走左转就能看到挂号处。

_____

21. 您需要看泌尿科医生。

_____

22. 我会将您带到内分泌科。

_____

23. 请先填写《初诊病人登记表》。

_____

24. 您需要有我院的就诊卡。

_____

25. 你可以提前一周预约。

_____

26. 你可以直接窗口预约,也可以通过电话、短信或网络等方式预约。

_____

- **Fill in the blanks to complete the sentences.**

Dialogue One

Doctor：Hello! Can I _____ you?

医生：你好，我能帮助你吗？

Patient：Hello, doctor! _____ you tell _____ where the _____ is?

病人：你好，医生，你能告诉我地铁站怎么走吗？

Doctor：You need to _____ a bus or a taxi to get to the subway _____.

医生：你需要坐公交车或的士到地铁站。

Patient：Oh, is it quite far _____ here?

病人：哦，离这里很远吗？

Doctor：Yes, it is. To take a bus, you need to go out of the hospital to the _____ road, and _____ the road. The bus stop is _____ your left. You will need to take the No. 3 bus.

医生：是的，如果坐公交车，你需要出医院到主路上去，然后过马路。公交站在你的左手边，你需要坐3路公交车。

Patient：How _____ will it take me to _____ to the subway?

病人：坐到地铁站需要多长时间？

Doctor：It _____ about 15 minutes.

医生：大约15分钟。

Patient：OK! Where _____ I take a taxi then?

病人：好的。在哪里乘坐出租车呢？

Doctor：Go _____ this door and walk _____ to the main road. There are a lot of taxis _____ there.

医生：穿过这个门，一直走到主路。那里有很多出租车在等待。

Patient：That's great! Thanks!

病人：太好了，谢谢！

Dialogue Two

Patient：Good morning.

病人：早晨好！

Nurse：Good morning. Do you want to _____ a doctor?

护士：早晨好！你是来看医生吗？

Patient：Yes，I have a _____ these days.

病人：对，这些天来我有些头痛。

Nurse：The first thing you should do is to _____ in the registration office.

护士：你先去挂号处挂个号。

Patient：Which _____ should I register with?

病人：我应该挂哪个科的号呢？

Nurse：You should see a _____ first. If _____ , the doctor will refer you to the _____ .

护士：你可以先去神经科看一看，如果有必要的话医生会让你去内科的。

Patient：Where is the registration office?

病人：挂号处在什么地方？

Nurse：Go straight _____ , and then turn left. The registration office is on the third floor. You can _____ the elevator at the _____ .

护士：直接往前走，然后左转，挂号处在三楼。你可以在拐角处乘坐电梯。

Dialogue Three

Patient：Hello，the doctor wanted me to do these exams. I am _____ where all these _____ are. Would you _____ pointing out the _____ for me?

病人：你好，医生让我做这些检查，但我不知道这个检查在哪里做。你能告诉我如何走吗？

Nurse：I would be happy to explain it to you. Please show me the exam application _____ .

护士：很乐意为您服务。请您把检查申请单给我看看。

Patient：Well，here it is.

病人：好的，在这。

Nurse：First，go _____ ahead. You'll find the _____ and you can _____ for all your applications there. Next，go to the _____ room for your ultrasound test on this floor. After that go _____ to the second floor for your CT in the _____ Department. Finally, go to the first floor to take the _____ test in the lab of _____ .

护士:首先,您一直往前走,到收费处交检查费。接下来到本层超声室做超声检查,做完后下到二楼放射科做CT,最后去一楼的化验室抽血化验。

Part Four

Other Structures

1. Excuse me, can/could you tell me which is the way to ... , (please)?
   打扰,请问你能告诉我去……的路吗?

2. Excuse me, could/can you tell me how to get/go to ... , (please)?
   打扰,请问你能告诉我怎么去……吗?

3. Excuse me, would you mind telling me the way to ... ?
   打扰,请问你能告诉我去……的路吗?

4. Excuse me, can you direct me to ... ?
   打扰,请问你能帮我指一下去……的路吗?

5. Excuse me, I wonder if you could do me a favor. I'm looking for ...
   打扰,你能帮我个忙吗? 我正在找……

6. Excuse me, how can I get to ... ?
   打扰,请问你能告诉我如何去……?

7. It's over there.
   在那边。

8. It's behind the ...
   在……后面。

9. It's next to the ...
   在……旁边。

10. It's across from ...
    在……对面。

11. It's in front of the ...
    它就在……前面。

12. It's near the ...

它在……附近。

13. It's on the right/left of the ...

它在……右/左边。

14. It's outside the ...

它在……外面。

15. It's on the other side of the ...

它在……对面。

16. in the east/west/south/north of ...

在……的东/南/西/北方

17. be far from

距离某处很远

18. go up/down

向上（北）/向下（南）

19. go back

向回走

20. go east/west/south/north

向东/西/南/北

21. go on/along ... till you meet ...

沿……一直走，直到

22. on the corner of A street and B street

在 A 和 B 街交汇的拐角处

23. in the corner of ...

在……的角落里

24. go straight across/to/through

径直走过/向/过

25. Walk along this road/street.

沿着这条路/街走。

26. It's about ... meters from here.

距离这里大约……米。

27. Take the ... turning on the left/right.

在第……个转弯处左/右转。

28. It's about ... meters along on the right/left.

沿右边/左边大约……米。

29. Walk on and turn left/right.

继续走再向左/右转。

30. Cross the street and go ahead.

过马路,一直往前走。

31. It'll take you no more than ten minutes to walk there.

用不了 10 分钟你就走到那儿了。

32. You're going in the opposite direction.

你方向走错了。

33. Go straight on,then turn left/right at the first/second crossing.

一直走,在第一/二个十字路口向左/右拐。

34. Go straight ahead about ... meters.

往前一直走……米。

35. Keep going until you see a ... on your left.

继续往前走,一直走到左边有……

36. Keep straight on for two blocks.

一直往前走,走过两条马路。

37. Walk one block east.

朝东走过一个街区。

38. Take the first turning on the left.

在第一个拐弯处向左拐。

39. Just follow this street two blocks.

沿着这条街走过两个街区就到。

40. It's just around the corner.

就在拐角处。

41. It's not far from here.

离这儿不远。

42. It's at the end of the street.

在这条街的尽头。

43. Turn right/left at the traffic lights. You'll find the ... on the right/left.

在交通灯右/左转，你会发现……在右/左边。

44. Go on until you reach the end of the road/street. You'll see the ... in front of you.

继续走一直到路/街的尽头，你就会看到……在你的面前。

Part Five

Supplementary Reading: Beyond the Handshake—How People Greet Each Other around the World

Here are 9 different ways to politely say hello in different countries and cultures—some of which don't involve any touching at all.

In many Western countries, a handshake is considered a warm, respectful greeting when meeting strangers or kicking off business meetings. But in other places in the world, not so much. Taking the time to learn how locals meet and greet is the first step to making a meaningful connection no matter where you are. From bumping noses in Qatar to bowing in Laos, here are 9 ways people greet each other in different countries and cultures. (Some of these gestures can be made without touching, which is especially helpful if you're currently opting for no-contact salutes to prevent the spread of coronavirus.)

1. Bump noses: *Qatar, Yemen, Oman, United Arab Emirates*

Want to demonstrate that you view a potential business contact as a peer. Forget shaking hands; instead, bring your nose in for a few friendly taps. Just remember: Sniffing isn't part of the equation.

2. Air kiss on the cheek: *France, Italy, Spain, Portugal, Latin America, Ukraine, and Québec, Canada, etc.*

In Argentina, Chile, Peru, Mexico, São Paulo (Brazil) and Colombia, one air kiss is standard, whereas in Spain, Portugal, Paraguay, Italy, and cities like Paris and Québec, it's two. In Russia and Ukraine, three is the norm, and in some parts of France, it's up to four air kisses on alternating cheeks. To add a little more confusion to the mix, there are some tricky gender and relationship rules, too. In all of the countries mentioned, women air kiss women, and in most of them, men air kiss women, but only in Argentina do men routinely brush cheeks with other men who aren't relatives or romantic partners.

3. Rub noses (and sometimes foreheads): *New Zealand*

If air kisses sound too intimate for your taste, try on hongi for size. This pressing together of forehead and nose is what New Zealand's indigenous Māori people call a "sharing of breath." The greeting signifies the sacred welcoming of a visitor into Māori culture and is used at pōwhiri (Māori welcoming ceremonies)—although the honor requires an invitation and isn't extended to everyone.

4. Shake hands: *Botswana, China, Germany, Zambia, Rwanda, and the Middle East*

A handshake isn't as simple as it seems when you take it on the road. In Middle Eastern countries, for example, handshakes involve the right hand only, where the left hand is considered unclean. Visitors to China will want to lighten their grip, while folks introducing themselves to Germans should know to stop after one firm downward yank.

Not sure what to do if your hand is dirty or wet? There are country-specific procedures in place for that, too. In Morocco, touch the back of your right hand to the back of the other person's right hand to complete the gesture. In Rwanda, grasp the other person's wrist, unless, of course, their hands are muddy too, in which case, just touch wrists to convey "hello." In Botswana, things are more complicated, even when hands are clean. The local handshake between two people entails multiple steps: Clasp right hands, shake up and down once, interlock thumbs, raise your arms to a right angle, grasp hands again, then release to a relaxed "shake" position before letting the other person's hand go.

5. Clap your hands: *Zimbabwe and Mozambique*

There's something kind of nice about applause as part of a hello, isn't there? In Zimbabwe, the clapping of hands comes after folks shake in a call and answer style—the first person claps once, and the second person twice, in response. Just be careful how you slap those palms together. Men clap with fingers and palms aligned, and women with their hands at an angle. In northern Mozambique, people also clap, but three times before they say "moni" (hello).

6. Put your hand on your heart: *Malaysia*

It's very formal, but this traditional Malaysian greeting has a particularly lovely sentiment behind it. Take the opposite person's hand lightly in yours. Then, release the other person's hand and bring your own hand to your chest and nod slightly to symbolize goodwill and an open heart. It's polite for the other person to return the gesture. Note that men should wait for local women to extend a hand, and if they don't, a man should put a hand on his chest and give a slight nod.

7. Bow: *Cambodia, India, Nepal, Laos, Thailand, and Japan*

When it comes to bowing, the question isn't just when to take a bow, it's how to do it. In India, Nepal, Cambodia, Laos, and Thailand, press your palms together in an upward-pointing prayer position at heart level or higher, then bend your head slightly forward to take a bow. In India and Nepal, you might hear the phrase "namaste" uttered during this greeting; the Sanskrit term translates to "bend or bow to you," and is considered a sign of respect and gratitude.

In Thailand, taking a bow is referred to as the wai, and the higher you place your hands, the more respect you're showing. In Japan, on the other hand, a deeper bow indicates a higher level of respect (90 degrees is the max) and prayer hands aren't used. Men bow with their hands at their sides, and women with their hands on their thighs. Among the younger generations, a head bow (like a nod, but more pronounced) is becoming the new norm.

8. Sniff faces: *Greenland and Tuvalu* (*Oceania*)

There's nothing quite like the smell of someone you love or someone you've just met. In Greenland, kunik, the Inuit tradition of placing your nose and upper lip against someone's cheek or forehead and sniffing, is limited to very close relationships. But on the South Pacific island of Tuvalu, pressing cheeks together and taking a deep breath is still part of a traditional Polynesian welcome for visitors.

9. Revere your elders: *Asia and Africa*

Throughout Asia and Africa, honoring your elders is a given. This means greeting seniors and older folks before younger people and always using culture-specific titles and terms of respect upon first meeting. In the Philippines, locals have a particularly unique way of showing their reverence. They take an older person's hand and press it gently to their foreheads. In India, locals touch older people's feet as a show of respect. In Liberia, as well as among members of the Yoruba people in Nigeria, young people drop to one or both knees to honor their elders.

Part Six
Conversational English Functions

- Opinions 观点

1. Asking for Opinions

What's your opinion of ... ?

What do you think of/about ... ?

What's your position on ... ?

What do you reckon about ... ?

How do you like ... ?

2. Giving Opinions

I'd like to point out that ...

In my opinion, ...

As far as I'm concerned, we should ...

From my point of view, I think that ...

Personally/Frankly speaking, I think that ...

I reckon that ...

If you ask me, I can tell you that ...

I'd say that ...

The point is that ...

As I see it, ...

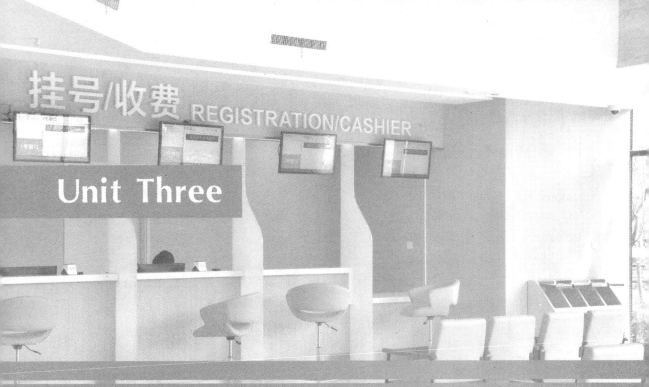

Unit Three

Dealing with Complaints
处理投诉

Learning Objectives

熟悉与投诉相关的词汇及表达

掌握处理投诉相关的句型结构

了解处理投诉的方式及技巧

Outline

Part One   Words and Expressions

Part Two   Model Dialogues

Part Three   Exercises

Part Four   Other Structures

Part Five   Supplementary Reading: How to Handle
              Patient Complaints

Part Six   Conversational English Functions
              • Repetition and Clarification

✓音、视频资源

✓参考答案

✓学术探讨

Part One

Words and Expressions

投诉	complain v. /	情况	situation
	complaint n.	误会	misunderstanding
问题的	problematic	愤怒	indignation
预期	expectation	描述	description
坚持	adhere	理解	comprehension
意见	opinion		

Part Two

Model Dialogues

Dialogue One

Patient：**I'm afraid I have to make a complaint.** Could you tell me when the doctor is coming? I have been waiting for 2 hours.

病人：我要投诉。你能告诉我医生什么时候来吗？我已经等了两个小时了。

Nurse：**I'm sorry to hear that.** I'm sure the doctor has been held up. I will go and check for you and let you know when he will be coming. I'm sorry you have waited so long.

护士：很抱歉听到这个消息。我确定医生是被什么事耽搁了。我去核实一下然后告诉你他什么时候来，抱歉让你等了那么长时间。

Patient：Thank you.

病人：谢谢。

Dialogue Two

Patient：Do I need to stay in hospital any longer? **I'm upset with** staying here. I'd rather go home.

病人：我还需要继续住院吗？我感到不安，我想回家。

Doctor：**I understand your feeling**，but it will be better if you stay for another day.

医生：我理解你的感受，不过在这多待一天康复效果会更好。

Patient：**I hate to say this**，but I feel I would be better off if I go home now. What do you have to do to me that I have to stay longer?

病人：我不想这样说，但我认为回家我会好得更快。你们将给我做什么以至于我必须再待更长的时间？

Doctor：**I hear what you are saying**，but we would prefer that you stay another day so that we are absolutely sure that you are better with no fever.

医生：我明白你的意思。但我们真的希望你能多待一天，以便于我们完全确认你已经好转不再发烧。

Dialogue Three

Nurse：Good morning. **This is Doctor Grant's office. This is Nurse Wang speaking.** What can I do for you?

护士：早上好，这里是 Grant 医生的办公室。我是王护士，有什么需要帮忙的吗？

Patient：Yes，this is Mrs. Stan. I'd like to make an appointment to see the doctor this week.

病人：我是 Stan 太太。我想预约本周看病。

Nurse：Well，let's see. I'm afraid Dr. Grant is fully engaged on Monday and Tuesday.

护士：好的。恐怕 Grant 医生本周星期一和星期二都已经约满了。

Patient：How about Thursday?

病人：星期四怎么样？

Nurse：Sorry，but I have to say he is also occupied on Thursday. So，will Wednesday be OK for you，Mrs. Stan?

护士：抱歉，星期四也已经约满了。Stan 太太，星期三您方便吗？

Patient：I have to work on Wednesday. By the way，is Dr. Grant available on Saturday?

病人：星期三我得上班。顺便问下，Grant 医生星期六有空吗？

Nurse：I'm afraid the office is closed on weekend.

护士：我们周末不上班。

Patient：Well，how about Friday?

病人：那么星期五如何？

Nurse：Friday. Let me check. Oh，good. Dr. Grant will be available on Friday afternoon this week.

护士：让我查一下。太好了，Grant 医生本周五下午有空。

Patient：That's fine. Thank you，I'll come then.

病人：太好了。谢谢你。到时我会来的。

Useful Structures

1. I'm afraid I have to make a complaint.

   我想我要投诉。

2. I'm sorry to hear that.

   很抱歉听到这个消息。

3. I'm upset with ...

   我对……感到不安。

4. I understand your feeling.

   我理解你的感受。

5. I hate to say this，but ...

   我不想这样说，但是……

6. This is Doctor Grant's office. This is Nurse Wang speaking.

   这里是 Grant 医生的办公室。我是王护士。

Part Three

Exercises

- Put the following sentences or expressions into English.

  1. 投诉　_____
  2. 误会　_____
  3. 愤怒　_____
  4. 意见　_____
  5. 情况　_____
  6. 预期　_____
  7. 描述　_____
  8. 理解　_____
  9. 我想要投诉。

  _____

  10. 能告诉我医生什么时候来吗?

  _____

  11. 我理解你的感受。

  _____

  12. 我想可能是有些误会。

  _____

  13. 对此我非常抱歉。

  _____

- Fill in the blanks to complete the dialogues.

Dialogue One

Patient: I have to _____. I have _____ in this room all morning and haven't seen one doctor.

病人:我要投诉。我整个早上都在这个房间等,没有见到一个医生。

Nurse: Really? I'm so _____. Please let me _____ out what has _____, and I'll come back and let you _____.

护士:真的吗? 对不起。我去了解一下,回来告诉你。

Dialogue Two

Patient：I hate to _____, but the nurse keeps coming and playing with the drip. Can you tell me what's _____ with it? Does she know what she is doing?

病人：我不想抱怨，可护士不停地来弄我的输液管，到底怎么回事？她知道她在做什么吗？

Nurse：I understand _____ you're feeling. I'm sure the nurse _____ what she is doing, but of course I will ask _____ nurse to have a _____ at it.

护士：我理解你的感受。我敢肯定护士知道她在干什么，当然我会找另外一个护士来看一下。

Patient：Thanks very much.

病人：非常感谢。

Dialogue Three

Patient：Doctor, I thought you said I _____ going to do an _____ this morning, but I haven't _____ one. In fact I haven't seen _____ since after breakfast.

病人：大夫，我记得你说我上午要做核磁共振检查，但我还没有做。实际上，早饭过后我再也没有看到任何（医务）人员。

Nurse：I'm _____ there _____ to be a _____. Your MRI is in the afternoon, and I'm sorry you haven't seen anyone _____ breakfast. I will go and see _____.

护士：恐怕这儿有误会。你的核磁检查安排在今天下午。对于早饭后没有人来照顾你我表示道歉，我将去调查原因。

Patient：OK. Thanks. What time this afternoon?

病人：好的，谢谢。下午什么时候？

Nurse：I'm afraid I can't tell you the _____ time, but it will be before 17：00. Is that OK?

护士：非常抱歉，我不能告诉你确切的时间，但是在5点之前，这样行吗？

Patient：I guess so.

病人：我觉得还行。

Nurse：Then I'll _____ you later.

护士：那一会见。

Patient：_____ a lot.

病人：非常感谢！

Part Four

Other Structures

1. I'm afraid there seems to be a misunderstanding.

   恐怕这儿有些误会。

2. Really? I am so sorry.

   真的吗？我很抱歉。

3. I am sure there must be a reason.

   我相信肯定是有原因的。

4. I do understand what you are saying.

   我确实理解你所说的一切。

5. I am sure there is a good explanation for ...

   对于……，我确信会有一个好的解释。

6. I am sorry you feel like that.

   你那样想，我感到很遗憾。

7. I hate to complain, but ...

   我不想抱怨，但是……

8. Excuse me, but there is a problem with ...

   对不起，……有问题。

9. Sorry to bother you, but I think there is something wrong with ...

   对不起打扰了，但我想……有问题。

10. I'm afraid there is a slight problem with ...

    恐怕这儿关于……有点小问题。

11. I'm sorry to say that ...

    我很抱歉地说……

12. I'm afraid I have to complain about ...

我恐怕要抱怨……

13. I can't say I feel happy about ...

我不能说对……感到高兴。

14. I'm not satisfied with ...

我对……不满意。

15. I'm dissatisfied with ...

我对……不满意。

16. I can't tell you how sorry I am.

我无法告诉你我有多抱歉。

17. I'm so/very/terribly/awfully sorry about this.

对这件事我非常抱歉。

18. I do apologize.

我道歉。

19. I assure you it won't happen again.

我保证这样的事不会再发生。

20. Thank you for bringing the matter to our attention.

感谢你让我们对这件事引起重视。

21. Sorry for having caused you so much trouble.

抱歉给你造成了这么多的麻烦。

22. Sorry，I didn't catch that. Did you say ... ?

抱歉，我没听明白你说的什么，你是说……吗？

23. I'm afraid I don't follow you. Could you repeat that please?

我恐怕没听明白，你能重说一遍吗？

24. I missed that. Would you mind repeating it?

我没听见，你介意重说一下吗？

25. I'm sorry, the line's bad—could you repeat what you just said?

对不起，线路不好，你能重复一下吗？

26. Please wait while I check that for you.

请稍等，我看一下。

27. One moment please while I double check on that for you.

稍微等,我帮你查一下。

28. I'm sorry, I can't hear you very well. Would you speak up a little, please?

对不起,我听不清,能大点声吗?

29. I am having difficulty hearing you. Please speak louder and speak directly into the mouthpiece of your telephone.

我听不清你的声音,能大点声并对准话筒说话吗?

30. Please speak a little more slowly.

请说慢一点。

31. She is talking on another line. Would you care to wait, or may I have her return your call?

她在接其他电话。你是等一下还是我让她一会给你回电话?

32. Would you like to hold, or would you prefer to leave a message?

你是稍等一下还是留下口信?

33. Could you put me through to ... Department, please?

能帮我转接……部门吗?

34. I'd like to speak with someone who deals with complaints.

我想和负责处理投诉的人通话。

35. Could you please return my call as soon as possible? My number is ... Thank you.

你能尽快给我回电吗? 我的电话是……,谢谢。

Part Five

Supplementary Reading: How to Handle Patient Complaints

It is impossible to make everyone happy all the time, and complaints are bound to happen within the medical field as often as in any other service industry. Disgruntled patients come with the territory and while you cannot eliminate potential issues completely, you can handle them in a way that benefits everyone. Follow these six steps for how to handle patient complaints that will leave patients feeling satisfied and heard.

1. <u>Listen to them.</u> As basic as it may sound, this is your first and most important step when dealing with an unhappy patient. Most of the time, people just

want to vent their frustrations to someone who is willing to listen. Be sure to give them your undivided attention, keep eye contact and truly hear what they have to say. Do not argue or pass blame, and be sure to control your emotions. Summarize what they have said to you so they know that you were listening. Remember that your ultimate goal is to retain this patient.

2. Acknowledge their feelings. Empathy is key when it comes to successfully handling patient complaints. Keep in mind that this person is a patient, he or she may not feel well or just received an unfortunate diagnosis. Put yourself in the patient's shoes and let him or her know that you understand his/her frustrations presented in this instance. Demonstrate to him/her that you care and that his or her feelings are valid.

3. Ask questions. Get as much information as possible. This will best help you and your staff figure out how to handle the complaint and avoid any issues that could arise in the future.

4. Explain and take action. Let the patient know that the complaint is being taken seriously and suggest solutions. Explain that it will be reviewed and discussed among the management. Inform the patient that you will follow up with him/her after the grievance has been thoroughly investigated. It is best practice to offer a time frame as to when the patient can expect a communication regarding the issue.

5. Conclude. Always thank patients for taking the time to speak with you and bringing the matter to your attention. Ensure they understand that their satisfaction is your number one priority.

6. Document complaints. Formally document any patient complaints, whether big or small. It is crucial that there is a protocol for handling these issues and ensuring grievances are followed up internally. If you promised to touch base with the patient, be sure to do so in a timely manner.

Patient complaints can be uncomfortable and frustrating, but try to stay positive. View complaints as an opportunity to learn and build upon that to provide an amazing office experience. Complaints are part of working in a medical field and should be expected. How you handle them and learn from them is what will set you apart from the competition.

Part Six

Conversational English Functions

• Repetition and Clarification 重复与澄清

1. Asking for Repetition and Clarification

I beg your pardon? /Pardon?

Would you mind repeating that?

Would you please repeat it?

I'm lost. I didn't catch the last part.

Sorry. I didn't hear what you said.

I'm sorry, but I didn't follow you.

Could you say that again?

I'm afraid I didn't understand what you just said.

I'm sorry, I don't quite understand what you mean by ...

I didn't quite follow what you were saying about ...

I'm sorry, but could you explain what you mean by ...

I don't quite see what you mean, I'm afraid.

I'm afraid I'm not really clear about what you mean by ...

I don't quite see what you're getting at.

Sorry, but I don't quite understand with what you said. Does it mean that ... ?

Can I get one thing clear? You think ... , don't you?

2. Giving Clarification

What I mean to say was ...

What I mean by ...

I guess what I was trying to say was ...

Well, the point I'm trying to make is that ...

Let me put it another way ...

Sorry，let me explain ...

That's not quite what I mean ...

Well，what I'm trying to say is that ...

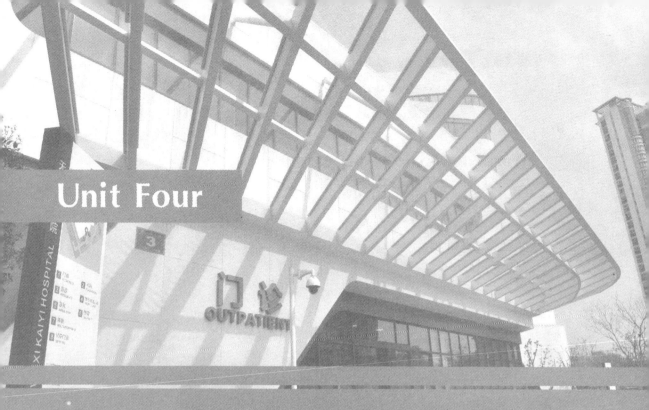

Unit Four

Inquiry—Diseases and Symptoms Ⅰ
问诊——疾病及症状（1）

Learning Objectives

熟悉身体部位及疼痛相关的词汇及表达

掌握问诊中与描述发病部位、时间及疼痛相关的句型结构

了解医患沟通技巧

Outline

✓音、视频资源

✓参考答案

✓学术探讨

Part One

Words and Expressions

下颚	jaw	肩	shoulder
颈	neck	腋窝	armpit
上臂	upper arm	背	back
肘	elbow	臀	buttock
手腕	wrist	小腿	calf
大腿	thigh	腿	leg
胸	chest	胃/腹部	stomach/tummy/abdomen
乳房	breast		
腹股沟	groin/inguen	肚脐	navel，belly button
膝盖	knee	脚后跟	heel
疼痛的	aching	疼痛	get/have/catch a pain
锐痛	sharp pain	抽痛	throbbing pain
压痛	tenderness	钝痛	dull pain
反跳触痛	rebound tenderness	刺痛	stabbing pain
绞痛	colicky pain	灼痛	burning pain
痉挛痛	crampy pain	僵硬的	stiff
肿胀的	swollen		

Part Two

Model Dialogues

Pain in Knees 膝盖疼痛

Doctor：**How can I help you**，Mr. Jones?

医生：琼斯先生，我能帮你什么吗?

Patient：I get a pain in my knees.

病人：我的膝盖疼痛。

Doctor：**What kind of pain do you feel**?

医生：你觉得是哪种疼痛？

Patient：It feels like a dull pain.

病人：感觉隐隐作痛。

Doctor：**Does it hurt when you press your knees**?

医生：当你按压膝盖时，感到疼痛吗？

Patient：Yes，it gets worse.

病人：是的，疼痛加剧。

Doctor：**How bad is it**?

医生：疼痛有多严重？

Patient：I think it seriously affects my walking.

病人：我觉得疼痛严重影响了我的行走。

Doctor：**When did the pain start**?

医生：疼痛什么时候开始的？

Patient：It began last month.

病人：自上月开始。

Doctor：**Did it happen suddenly or gradually**?

医生：疼痛是突然发生还是逐渐发生的？

Patient：It happened suddenly.

病人：疼痛是突然发生的。

Doctor：**Do you have it all the time or does it come and go**?

医生：持续疼痛还是间歇疼痛？

Patient：I feel the pain all the time.

病人：我一直感觉疼痛。

Doctor：**Does the pain go anywhere else**?

医生：疼痛会转移吗？

Patient：It doesn't seem to move.

病人：貌似不会转移。

Doctor：**Do you have any other problems related to the pain**?

医生：还有其他与疼痛相关的问题吗？

Patient：My knees are swollen and a little stiff.

病人：我的膝盖肿胀，有点僵硬。

Doctor：I see.

医生：我了解了。

Headache 头痛

Doctor：**What's wrong with you**?

医生：你怎么了？

Patient：I have a headache.

病人：我头疼。

Doctor：**Can you point out the painful area**?

医生：你能指出疼痛的部位吗？

Patient：It seems to be on the left side of my head.

病人：好像是我的左脑疼。

Doctor：**Could you describe the pain**?

医生：你可以描述一下疼痛吗？

Patient：It feels like a sharp pain.

病人：感觉像锐痛。

Doctor：**When did this happen**?

医生：疼痛何时发生的？

Patient：It happened several days ago.

病人：几天前。

Doctor：**How long does the headache last**?

医生：头痛持续多久？

Patient：It varies; it can be between half an hour and four or five hours.

病人：疼痛持续时间不等，在半小时和四五个小时之间。

Doctor：**Is it always just in that spot**?

医生：总是那里疼吗？

Patient：No, sometimes it moves to the right side.

病人：不是，有时疼痛会转移到右边。

Doctor：**When you get the headache，does anything happen at the same time**?

医生：当你头疼时，还有其他症状同时发生吗?

Patient：Sometimes I feel dizzy and would like to vomit.

病人：有时，我感觉头晕，想吐。

Useful Structures

1. How can I help you?

   我能帮你什么吗?

2. What's wrong with you?

   你怎么了?

3. Can you point out the painful area?

   你能指出疼痛的部位吗?

4. What kind of pain do you feel?

   你觉得是哪种疼痛?

5. Could you describe the pain?

   你可以描述一下疼痛吗?

6. Does it hurt when you press your knees?

   当你按压膝盖时，感到疼痛吗?

7. How bad is it?

   疼痛有多严重?

8. When did the pain start?

   疼痛何时开始?

9. When did this happen?

   疼痛何时发生的?

10. How long does the headache last?

    头痛持续多久?

11. Did it happen suddenly or gradually?

    疼痛是突然发生还是逐渐发生的?

12. Do you have it all the time or does it come and go?

    持续疼痛还是间歇疼痛?

13. Does the pain go anywhere else?

疼痛会转移吗？

14. Is it always just in that spot?

总是那里疼吗？

15. Do you have any other problems related to the pain?

还有其他与疼痛相关的问题吗？

16. When you get the headache，does anything happen at the same time?

当你头疼时,还有其他症状吗？

Part Three

Exercises

• Put the following sentences or expressions into English.

1. 钝痛 _____ 2. 锐痛 _____

3. 腹部 _____ 4. 小腿 _____

5. 刺痛 _____ 6. 压痛 _____

7. 腋窝 _____ 8. 下颚 _____

9. 你能指出疼痛的部位吗？

_____

10. 你可以描述一下疼痛吗？

_____

11. 疼痛何时开始？

_____

12. 疼痛会转移吗？

_____

• The following questions are useful when asking a patient about his present condition. Match the questions that have the same meaning.

1. What can I do for you?
2. What's the pain like?
3. Did it start suddenly?
4. Is it always in that spot?
5. Does anything else happen at the same time?

A. Did your condition change without any warning?
B. Do you have any other symptom?
C. Does it move to another part of your body?
D. Could you describe the pain?
E. What's wrong with you?

• Fill in the blanks to complete the dialogue.

Doctor: What's the matter with you?

医生:你怎么了?

Patient: I feel feverish.

病人:我觉得有点发热。

Doctor: Have you taken your _____?

医生:你量过体温吗?

Patient: Yes, I took it at home. It was 39 ℃.

病人:是的,在家量过体温。体温是 39 ℃。

Doctor: When _____ _____ _____ _____?

医生:什么时候开始发热的?

Patient: The night before last.

病人:前晚。

Doctor: Do you have any other _____?

医生:你还有其他症状吗?

Patient: Yes, I catch a _____ in my _____.

病人:是的,我头疼。

Doctor: What _____ _____ _____ is that?

医生:何种疼痛?

Patient: It seems like _____ _____ _____.

病人：感觉像抽痛。

Doctor：Does the pain _____ _____ _____ _____ of the body?

医生：疼痛会转移到身体的其他部位吗？

Patient：No, it seems to be always in that spot.

病人：不会，疼痛总在那个部位。

Part Four

Other Structures

Main Site 发病部位

1. Where does it hurt?

   哪里疼？

2. Show me where it hurts.

   告诉我哪里疼。

3. Can you show me the painful area?

   你能指出疼痛部位吗？

4. Where is the pain?

   哪里疼？

5. Tell me where your pain is located.

   告诉我哪里疼。

6. Can you tell me where you feel the pain?

   你能告诉我哪里疼吗？

Radiation 疼痛扩散

1. Does it go anywhere else?

   它（疼痛）会转移到其他部位吗？

2. Does the pain spread to any other area?

   疼痛会蔓延到其他部位吗？

3. Does it move anywhere else?

它(疼痛)会转移到其他部位吗?

4. Does it affect any other parts of your body?

它会影响身体的其他部位吗?

5. Do you feel it anywhere else?

其他部位能感受到它(疼痛)吗?

Character 疼痛性质

1. What's the pain like?

何种疼痛?

2. What kind of pain do you feel?

你感到何种疼痛?

3. Can you describe the pain?

你能形容一下疼痛吗?

4. Is the pain constant or does it come and go?

疼痛是持续的还是间断的?

5. When you get the pain, is it steady, or does it change?

疼痛是稳定的还是会改变的?

6. Was it sharp, dull or aching?

锐痛,钝痛还是酸痛?

Time 发病时间

1. When did it start?

何时开始?

2. Did it start suddenly?

它是突然发生的吗?

3. Did it start gradually?

它是逐步发生的吗?

4. How long has it been bothering you?

它困扰您多久了?

5. How long have you had this pain?

你疼多久了?

6. How often do you get them?

你多久疼一次?

Part Five

Supplementary Reading: How to Explain Your Pain to a Doctor (Excerpt)

An experienced chiropractor has tips to help you get the care you need at your next appointment submitted by Dr. Michael J. Cooney, DC.

For more than three decades, I've been treating patients with acute and chronic pain from around the corner here in Rutherford, New Jersey to as far away as Australia and South Africa.

From our patient's first consultation to the last treatment office visit, the success of any pain treatment we prescribe is contingent upon us (the health care provider), accurately treating the root cause of your pain.

As the patient, precisely describing your acute pain or neuropathic pain is a "high stakes" conversation. I can read your medical history, referring doctor reports and lab results, but this is all secondary to understanding each patient's pain mechanics. It is absolutely essential that this is communicated to your pain management provider as accurately as possible.

For those battling "invisible pain" such as fibromyalgia, CRPS (complex regions pain syndrome), RSD (reflex sympathetic dystrophy), diabetic neuropathy or chronic pain after cancer treatment, accurately conveying the location, frequency and depth of the discomfort can be particularly challenging and emotionally taxing.

If you or a loved one are combatting short-term (acute) pain or a neuropathy (pain lasting 12 weeks or longer), I'd like to offer my own simple tools to help you accurately convey the unique characteristics of your pain so that the most effective treatment protocol can be set into motion.

You may wish to bring this article to your next doctor visit and go over each of the key pain description points I've outlined below.

I hope your doctor will ask you these questions, but if not, you can act as your own pain advocate and offer this information.

"Tell Me About Your Pain"

Based upon your medical records, we already know the cause of your pain (injury or disease).

Our goal is to eliminate or minimize this symptom so you can resume your highest quality of life possible.

Pain symptoms are personal, unique—and subjective. (What Joe describes as "unbearable pain" may be considered "pretty unpleasant pain" to Mike.) Over the years, I developed my own "pain diagnostic" conversation with patients to help my team and I understand what, where, when and how much pain patients are feeling. I've outlined key points below:

Timing Matters

This is key to a proper diagnosis. Don't assume we know you've battled this pain for a year, a month or a decade.

Spell it out:

1. I've had this pain for _____.

2. How frequently and how long does it last?

3. What ignites (flare) or lessens your pain and for how long?

Location, Location, Location

Where does it hurt? Doctors may instruct you to mark the area/s where your pain is concentrated. They may also ask you to note a difference between pain that is on the surface and pain that is under the surface.

This tool comes from the McGill Pain Questionnaire which includes other measurements, but the front and back of the unisex human figure are the most recognizable.

How Bad is Your Pain—A Measurement Tool

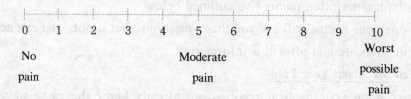

Most referring physicians, regardless of their medical specialty, use a simple 1 to 10 point pain scale, so I stick with this to keep everyone on the same page.

Simply stated, think about where your pain level falls the majority of the time—unless you experience extreme pain fluctuations.

No Pain

0—Pain-free

Manageable Pain

1—Pain is very mild, barely noticeable. Most of the time you don't think about it.

2—Minor pain. Annoying and may have occasional stronger twinges.

3—Pain is noticeable and distracting, however, you can get used to it and adapt.

Moderate Pain—Disrupts normal daily living activities

4—Moderate pain. If you are deeply involved in an activity, it can be ignored for a period of time, but is still distracting.

5—Moderately strong pain. It can't be ignored for more than a few minutes, but you still can manage to work or participate in some social activities.

6—Moderately strong pain that interferes with normal daily activities. Difficulty concentrating.

Severe Pain—Disabling; debilitating, reduces daily quality of life, cannot live independently

7—Severe pain that dominates your senses and significantly limits your ability to perform normal daily activities or maintain social relationships. Interferes with sleep.

8—Intense pain. Physical activity is severely limited. Conversing requires great effort.

9—Excruciating pain. Unable to converse. Crying out and/or moaning uncontrollably.

10—Unspeakable pain. Bedridden and possibly delirious. Mobility may be compromised.

"My Pain Feels Like ... "

Most of the time, patients experience one or two consistent pain "feelings" but some can experience a range of sensations.

The most common pain types are:

- Sharp stabbing pain
- Extreme heat or burning sensation
- Extreme cold
- Throbbing, "swollen," inflamed tissue
- Sensitivity to contact/touching
- Itching
- Numbness, tingling, pins and needles

Create a Pain Journal

I always encourage patients or their loved ones to document a week-long paincycle before they meet with their pain management, chiropractic or alternative medicine team. Also, jot down any treatments or actions that lessen or increase your discomfort. For example, perhaps you've found that hot showers or cold weather makes you feel worse, but Epsom salt baths or exercise makes the pain more manageable.

If you come prepared with all this information, your time with the doctor can be better spent focusing on next steps and a treatment plan, rather than a lengthy Q & A review of the information provided here.

More importantly, addressing these issues in advance will ensure your doctor receives up-to-date, higher quality information.

As a result, your case can be assessed more quickly and a pain management plan can be put into action to start reducing or eliminating your discomfort as quickly and effectively as possible.

Part Six

Conversational English Functions

- Apology 道歉

1. Apologizing

Excuse me (for my ...).

Pardon me.

I can't tell you how sorry I am.

I'm afraid I've brought you too much trouble.

I hope you will pardon me for my ...

I must make an apology for ...

I do beg your pardon (for ...).

May I offer you my profoundest/sincerest apologies (for ...)?

Please forgive me (for ...).

2. Responding to Apologies

Don't let it worry/distress you.

Don't think any more about it.

It doesn't matter at all.

Never mind. It doesn't really matter.

Please don't worry about that.

Please don't take it too hard.

Forget it.

No harm (done).

That's OK.

You're welcome.

Not in the least.

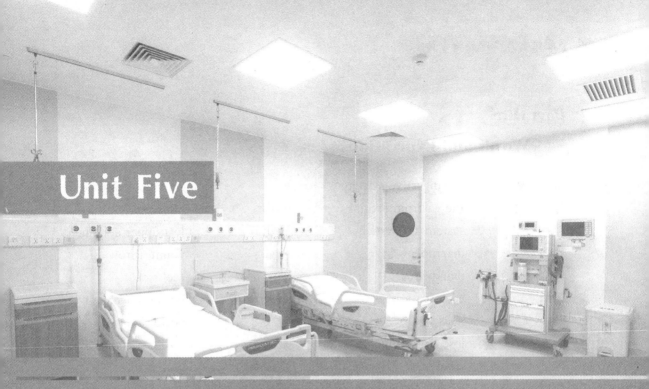

Unit Five

Inquiry—Diseases and Symptoms Ⅱ
问诊——疾病与症状(2)

Learning Objectives

熟悉常见疾病名称

掌握问诊中与病情发作、症状加重及缓解相关的句型结构

进一步掌握医患沟通技巧

Outline

✓音、视频资源

✓参考答案

✓学术探讨

Part One

Words and Expressions

消化系统	the digestive system		infectious diseases
胃肠系统	the gastrointestinal system/GI system	腹部	abdomen
		左上腹	left upper abdomen
腹泻	diarrhoea(英)/ diarrhea(美)	呕吐	vomit/throw up
		感觉恶心	feel sick
便秘	constipation	排便	bowel movement
恶心,反胃	nausea	排便习惯	bowel habit
失去胃口	lose one's appetite	肠鸣音	bowel sound
粪便	stool	胃溃疡	gastric ulcer
包块	mass	上呼吸道感染	upper respiratory tract infection
急性肠胃炎	acute gastroenteritis		
呼吸系统	the respiratory system	下呼吸道感染	lower respiratory tract infection
湿啰音	moist crackles/rale	咳嗽	cough
喘鸣	wheeze	痰	sputum/phlegm
疲劳,乏力	fatigue	咳嗽带痰	a productive cough/ a loose cough
寒战	shiver/rigor		
哮喘	asthma	痰中带血	blood-stained sputum(or phlegm)
病毒性肺炎	viral pneumonia		
胸膜炎	pleurisy	血痰	bloody sputum/ phlegm
非典型性肺炎	Severe Acute Respiratory Syndrome(SARS)		
		有痰的	productive
		无痰的	non-productive
中东呼吸综合征	Middle East Respiratory Syndrome(MERS)	咳嗽不带痰(干咳)	a non-productive cough/a dry cough
乙类传染病	category B	清痰/白痰	mucoid sputum/ phlegm

脓痰	purulent sputum/ phlegm	肺炎	pneumonia
泡沫痰	frothy sputum/ phlegm	支气管炎	bronchitis
锈色痰	rusty sputum/ phlegm	急性呼吸窘迫综合征	Acute Respiratory Distress Syndrome（ARDS）
发烧	fever		
胸闷	chest distress	禽流感病毒	avian influenza virus
出汗	sweating		
气短/呼吸困难	dyspnea/shortness of breath	2019 新型冠状病毒	COVID-19

Part Two

Model Dialogues

Abdominal Pain 腹痛

Doctor：**Do you feel any pain**?

医生：你觉得疼吗?

Patient：Yes，quite a bit.

病人：是的,很疼。

Doctor：**Could you show me the painful area**?

医生：你能指出疼痛的部位吗?

Patient：Right here.（The patient points to the left upper abdomen.）

病人：在这里。（病人指着自己的左上腹。）

Doctor：**Is it just always in that spot**?

医生：疼痛总是固定在这个部位吗?

Patient：No，sometimes it moves around to here.

病人：不是,有时会移到这里。

Doctor：**What kind of pain is it**?

医生：何种疼痛?

Patient：Well，it feels like a crampy pain.

病人：感觉像痉挛痛。

Doctor：**How long has this been going on**?

医生：这种情况持续多久了？

Patient：Since three days ago.

病人：从三天前开始。

Doctor：**Was there anything that seemed to cause this**?

医生：可能是什么原因导致疼痛发生？

Patient：I am not sure if it has anything to do with the barbecue I had several days ago.

病人：我不确定是否和我几天前吃的烧烤有关系。

Doctor：**Does anything else happen at the same time**?

医生：还有其他症状吗？

Patient：I feel sick and lose my appetite.

病人：感觉恶心，没有胃口。

Doctor：**Have you vomited**?

医生：呕吐了吗？

Patient：No.

病人：没有。

Doctor：**Have you noticed any change of bowel habit**? In other words, **are you going to the toilet more often than normal**?

医生：排便习惯发生改变了吗？换句话说，排便次数有所增多吗？

Patient：Yes, more often than normal. About four times a day on average.

病人：是的，排便次数有所增多，平均大概一天四次。

Doctor：**Are your stools hard or loose**?

医生：硬便还是稀便？

Patient：My stools are loose.

病人：稀便。

Doctor：**Is there any blood in your stools**?

医生：大便里有血吗？

Patient：No.

病人：没有。

Cough 咳嗽

Doctor：What's the problem?

医生：哪里不舒服?

Patient：I cough a lot, especially at night.

病人：我咳嗽厉害,尤其在晚上。

Doctor：**Do you cough up any phlegm**?

医生：咳痰吗?

Patient：Yes.

病人：是的。

Doctor：**Is it thick and sticky**?

医生：是黏稠的浓痰吗?

Patient：Yes, it is sticky and feels like jelly.

病人：是的,痰液黏稠,呈胶状。

Doctor：**What color is it**?

医生：痰是什么颜色?

Patient：Usually yellow.

病人：通常是黄色。

Doctor：**Have you ever noticed any blood in it**?

医生：你注意到痰中有血吗?

Patient：No, there is no blood in it.

病人：痰中没有血。

Doctor：**Are there any problems with your breathing**?

医生：呼吸有什么问题吗?

Patient：Yes, I find it a little difficult to breathe when I go up the stairs.

病人：上楼时,呼吸有点困难。

Doctor：**When did the cough start**?

医生：何时开始咳嗽?

Patient：About one week ago.

病人：一周前。

Doctor：**How often do you cough**?

医生：多久咳嗽一次？

Patient：About ten to twenty times a day.

病人：每天大约十到二十次。

Doctor：**Does anything relieve the symptom or make it worse**?

医生：有什么能缓解咳嗽症状或有什么会使咳嗽症状加重呢？

Patient：Nothing seems to relieve my cough. I took some cough medicine，but it didn't help much.

病人：似乎没有什么可以减轻我的症状。我吃了一些咳嗽药，但没有多大作用。

Doctor：I see. **Do you have any other symptoms**?

医生：了解了。你还有其他症状吗？

Patient：I feel fatigue and have a pain in my chest. When I cough，the pain gets worse.

病人：我感觉乏力，胸部疼痛。咳嗽时，疼痛加剧。

Useful Structures

1. Do you feel any pain?

   你觉得疼吗？

2. Could you show me the painful area?

   你能指出疼痛的部位吗？

3. Is it just always in that spot?

   疼痛总是固定在这个部位吗？

4. What kind of pain is it?

   何种疼痛？

5. How long has this been going on?

   这种情况持续多久了？

6. Was there anything that seemed to cause this?

   可能是什么原因导致这（疼痛）发生呢？

7. Does anything else happen at the same time?

   还有其他症状吗？

8. Have you vomited?

你呕吐了吗？

9. Have you noticed any change of bowel habit?

排便习惯发生改变了吗？

10. Are you going to the toilet more often than normal?

排便次数有所增多吗？

11. Are the stools hard or loose?

硬便还是稀便？

12. Is there any blood in your stools?

大便里有血吗？

13. Do you cough up any phlegm?

咳痰吗？

14. Is it (the phlegm) thick and sticky?

是黏稠的浓痰吗？

15. What colour is (the phlegm)...?

（痰）是什么颜色？

16. Have you ever noticed any blood in it?

你注意到痰中有血吗？

17. Are there any problems with your breathing?

呼吸有什么问题吗？

18. When did the cough start?

何时开始咳嗽？

19. How often do you cough?

多久咳嗽一次？

20. Does anything relieve the symptom or make it worse?

有什么能缓解咳嗽症状或有什么事会使咳嗽症状加重呢？

21. Do you have any other symptoms?

你还有其他症状吗？

Part Three
Exercises

- Fill in the blanks to complete the dialogue.

Doctor：So _____ me _____ your problem is.

医生：那么,请告诉我你哪里不舒服。

Patient：I have _____ a few times and I _____ nauseous though I don't know _____.

病人：我呕吐了几次,感到恶心,但是不知道什么原因。

Doctor：Did you vomit _____ _____?

医生：你吐的是未消化的食物吗?

Patient：Not really.

病人：不完全是。

Doctor：Have you _____ _____ that might have _____ you feel this _____?

医生：你是否吃了什么东西才会这样?

Patient：No, I don't think so.

病人：我想没有。

Doctor：Do you have any other _____? Such as _____ pain or _____?

医生：你还有其他症状吗? 例如腹痛或头痛?

Patient：Yes, I have a pain in my _____.

病人：我的腹部疼痛。

- Match the following expressions with the given words.

a productive cough	vomit	rigor	fatigue	dyspnea
a non-productive cough	nausea	phlegm	fever	symptom

1. throw up _____　　2. tiredness _____

3. shiver _____　　4. complaint _____

5. sputum _____   6. feel sick _____

7. have a temperature _____   8. a dry cough _____

9. a loose cough _____   10. shortness of breath _____

Part Four

Other Structures

Aggravating Factors 病情加重因素

1. Does anything make it worse?
   有什么会使它加重？

2. Is there anything else that affects it?
   还有其他影响吗？

Relieving Factors 病情缓解因素

1. Does anything make them better?
   有什么会使它好转？

2. What do you do to get more comfortable?
   你会做些什么让自己感觉更舒服？

3. Does lying quietly in bed help you?
   安静地躺在床上有帮助吗？

4. Does rest help?
   休息有用么？

5. Does aspirin help the headache?
   阿司匹林能缓解头痛么？

6. Does eating make it better?
   吃东西会缓解么？

Precipitating Factors 病情诱发因素

1. Does anything bring them on?

是什么导致它们（疾病）发生？

2. What makes it worse?

什么情况下会加重？

3. What seems to bring on the pain?

什么会引起疼痛？

4. Have you noticed that it occurs at a certain time of day?

你有没有留意过是否会在某个固定时间段发生？

5. Is there anything else besides exercise that makes it worse?

除了运动之外，还有什么会让症状更糟？

6. Does exercise increase the shortness of breath?

运动会加剧呼吸急促么？

7. Does stress precipitate the pain?

压力会加剧疼痛么？

Accompanying Symptoms 伴随症状

1. Do you have any other problems related to the pain?

你还有与该疼痛相关的其他症状吗？

2. Do you feel anything else wrong when it's there?

你还感觉哪里不舒服？

3. Does any symptoms happen at the same time?

有与此同时发生的症状吗？

4. Do you have any other symptoms?

你还有其他症状么？

5. Do you ever have nausea with the pain?

你是否有过疼痛伴恶心？

6. Have you noticed other changes that happen when you start to sweat?

你有没有在开始出汗的时候发现身体其他方面的改变呢？

7. Before you get the headache，do you ever experience a strange taste or smell?

你在发生头疼之前，是否曾尝到或闻到什么奇怪的东西？

Part Five

Supplementary Reading: Deciding When to See a Doctor

Should I go to the doctor? Most of us have asked that question at one time or another. Whether it's a bad cold, a funny-looking mole, or that nagging pain that just won't get away, it can be hard to know when you should be seen by a doctor. There are no set rules that tell you when to go or when to wait. But some general guidelines might help you the next time you're trying to decide.

Path to improved health

Below are some common illnesses and problems we may deal with from time to time. Many of them can be managed at home. But sometimes they can progress or change, and then it's best if they are addressed by a doctor. If you aren't sure what to do, call your doctor. He or she, or even a nurse in the office, can tell you if you should make an appointment.

Common cold or flu

Many symptoms can be managed with plenty of rest, fluids, and over-the-counter medicine. But if you experience any of these symptoms, call your doctor:

- Painful swallowing(more than a sore or dry throat).
- Earache.
- A cough that lasts more than 2 or 3 weeks.
- Persistent or severe vomiting.
- A fever that doesn't go down or go away.
- Symptoms that last more than 10 days or get worse instead of better.

Diarrhea

Occasional diarrhea is not uncommon. It is usually harmless and doesn't mean something is wrong. But there are signs to look for that could indicate a problem. These include:

- Diarrhea that lasts more than 3 days.
- Black, tarry stools.

- Blood in your stool.

- Severe abdominal pain.

- Signs of dehydration (very dry mouth or skin, fatigue, decreased urination, confusion or irritability).

Headache

We all get headaches every once in a while. They usually go away with rest or over-the-counter medicine. But headache can also be a sign of a serious condition, such as stroke or meningitis. If you have a high fever, stiff neck, confusion, or trouble speaking or walking along with a headache, go to the emergency room. If you have any of the following, schedule an appointment with your doctor:

- Headaches that are different than normal (more often or more severe).

- Headaches that get worse or don't get better after taking over-the-counter medicine.

- Headaches that keep you from working, sleeping, or participating in activities.

Digestive issues

Digestive issues can include problems in the upper digestive tract (esophagus and stomach), as well as the lower tract (intestines). If you experience any of the following, call your doctor:

- Feeling like food is caught in your throat or chest.

- Heartburn that doesn't go away, gets worse, or doesn't get better with medicine.

- Difficult or painful swallowing.

- Hoarseness or sore throat that doesn't go away.

- Nausea that won't go away.

- Vomiting blood or bile (green).

- Severe or persistent abdominal pain.

- Constipation or diarrhea that won't go away.

- Stools that are black or bloody.

Back pain

Most back pain will go away in a few weeks without treatment. It often gets better by using over-the-counter medicine. You can also apply heat or cold to the area that hurts. But sometimes it is a sign of a problem. Call your doctor if you experience:

- Constant pain.
- Pain that spreads down one or both legs, especially if it goes past your knee.
- Pain with weakness, numbness, or tingling in one or both legs.
- Pain plus unexplained weight loss.
- Pain with swelling or redness on your back.
- Pain with a fever.

Head injury

Getting a bump on the head could be minor. But it also could cause a concussion. Look for these signs of concussion and call your doctor if you have any of them after hitting your head:

- Dizziness and balance problems.
- Nausea and vomiting.
- Confusion.
- Concentration and memory problems.
- Feeling sluggish or foggy.
- Sensitivity to light or noise.
- Sleep problems.
- Mood changes.

Menstrual problems

A woman's monthly period can have a big impact on her life, especially if there are problems. Call your doctor if you are experiencing any of these symptoms:

- Period suddenly becomes irregular.
- No period in 3 months or more.
- Bleeding between periods.
- A period that lasts much longer than usual or is much heavier than usual.
- Severe or disabling cramps.

Mental health issues

Mental health is an important part of our overall health and should never be ignored. Having issues with mental health is also very common and treatable. Call your doctor if you are experiencing any of these signs of trouble with your mental health.

- Feelings of depression or sadness that don't go away.
- Feeling extreme highs and lows.
- Having excessive fear, worry, or anxiety.
- Withdrawing from social interactions.
- Changes in eating or sleeping.
- Inability to cope with daily problems.
- Delusions or hallucinations.
- Substance abuse.
- Thoughts of hurting yourself or others.

Other symptoms

Some symptoms are hard to categorize, but they are still important to take note of. The following symptoms could be signs of a problem that may need to be addressed by a doctor:

- Dizziness or feeling like you are going to faint.
- Shortness of breath.
- Heart palpitations.
- Unexplained weight loss.
- Fatigue that won't go away.
- Severe sweating, especially cold sweats.
- Swelling in the ankles or legs.
- Rash along with a fever (38 ℃ or higher).
- A new or changing mole or other skin change that concerns you.
- Things to consider.

Most people don't go to the doctor unless they are sick or they have a problem. But you should start by seeing your doctor when you're well. By seeing your doctor routinely, you can stay on top of your health. He or she can provide preventive health screenings and monitor your health over time. This allows them to catch diseases early and help you manage them before they progress into more serious conditions.

Part Six

Conversational English Functions

• Approval and Disapproval 赞成与不赞成

Are you in favour of his opinion?

Do you think it's a good idea?

Are you for ... ?

Does that meet your approval?

What is your attitude towards ... ?

Could I ask for your reaction to ... ?

Do you approve of ... ?

... has your approval, hasn't it?

That's what I had in mind.

How wise of you!

I think I would go along with that.

I'm sure you're right.

That's a good idea!

That's exactly my opinion.

I absolutely/entirely/certainly approve of ...

Suits me fine.

You've got something there.

There's something in what he says.

I really don't approve of ...

I don't suppose that's right, really.

Do you honestly feel that's reasonable?

I'm not so sure ... , you know.

I think that's dreadful!

That's quite wrong.

Are you out of your mind?

Surely not!

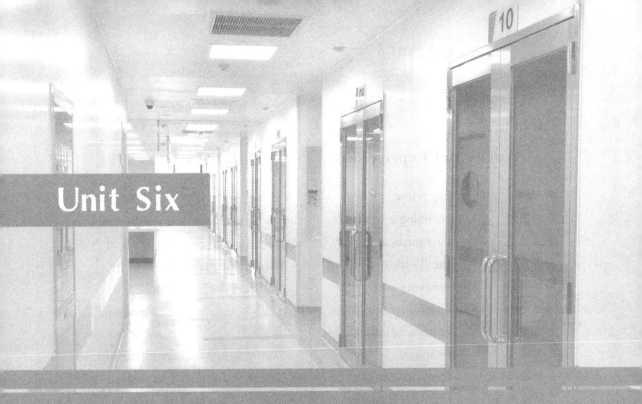

Unit Six

Inquiry—Diseases and Symptoms Ⅲ
问诊——疾病与症状（3）

Learning Objectives

熟悉与既往病史、职业史、家族史、社会史等相关的词汇及表达
掌握问诊中与既往病史、职业史、家族史、社会史等相关的句型结构
了解英文病史书写的相关内容

Outline

✓音、视频资源
✓参考答案
✓学术探讨

Part One

Words and Expressions

问诊	interview
病理原因	pathologic cause
既往病史	past medical history
家族史	family history
缓解因素	relieving factor
住院史	hospitalization
免疫接种	immunization
破伤风	tetanus
粪口途径	fecal-oral route
乙肝携带者	hepatitis B carrier
失眠	insomnia
阻塞型睡眠	obstructive sleep
呼吸暂停	apnea
非处方药物	over-the-counter medication
草药	herbal medication
健康维持	health maintenance
消遣性药物/消遣性毒品	recreational drug
家谱	pedigree/family chart
MMR 疫苗(麻疹、腮腺炎、风疹联合疫苗)	measles, mumps and rubella vaccine
吸烟包/年＝抽烟年数×每日抽烟包数	pack year(pack year＝ the number of years a patient has smoked × the number of packs per day)
来源及可信度	source and reliability
主诉	chief complaint
认知功能	cognitive function
加重因素	aggravating factor
过敏	allergy
免疫反应	allergic response
白喉	diphtheria
甲型/乙型肝炎	hepatitis A/B
随访剂量	follow-up dose
加强剂量	booster dose
嗜睡	somnolence
处方药物	prescription medication
物质滥用	substance abuse
睡眠规律	sleep pattern
职业和环境史	occupational and environmental history
直系亲属	immediate family member

Part Two

Model Dialogues

Doctor：**What seems to be the problem**，Mr. Smith?

医生：您遇到了什么问题,史密斯先生?

Patient：I've been having this chest pain for the past 6 months. In 2012, I had my first heart attack and admitted to hospital for 2 weeks.

病人：6个月来,我一直有胸部疼痛。2012年我经历了第一次心脏病发作,住院了2周。

Doctor：**How did you feel when you were discharged from the hospital**?

医生：出院时感觉怎么样?

Patient：I felt fine. Chest pain occurs no more. My doctor there had prescribed some pills for me and said I would be fine.

病人：我真觉得不错。胸部不再疼了。那边的医生给我开了一些药,说我不会有事的。

Doctor：Then what happened?

医生：然后发生了什么?

Patient：I went back to work after about 3 weeks. I really felt everything was back to normal!

病人：3周后我回到了工作岗位。我真的感觉一切恢复常态了!

Doctor：What kind of work do you do?

医生：你从事什么工作?

Patient：I'm a lawyer.

病人：我是一个律师。

Doctor：You told me that this was your first heart attack. Have you had others?

医生：你提到这是你的第一次心脏病发作。你还有其他的么?

Patient：Yes. Six months later，I had my second one.

病人：确实有。6个月之后,我第二次心脏病发作。

Doctor：What were you doing then?

医生：你当时在做什么？

Patient：Playing tennis.

病人：打网球。

Doctor：Did your doctor run any tests while you were in the hospital?

医生：你在医院有没有做过任何检查？

Patient：No. The doctor just gave me some pills to strengthen my heart and for the irregularity. It seems the pain never goes away.

病人：没有。医生只是给了我一些用来增强心肌和心律不齐的药物。我觉得疼痛始终存在。

Doctor：What's the pain like now?

医生：疼痛现在是什么样的？

Patient：It's an awful tightness. Right here.

病人：一种剧烈的紧缩感。就在这。

Doctor：When the pain occurs, does it restrict in certain body locations?

医生：当疼痛发生时，它只会局限在身体的某些部位么？

Patient：Yeah. It goes straight to my back and my right arm. The arm feels heavy when the pain occurs.

病人：会的。它会直达我的背部和我的右臂。疼痛发生时膀子会感到很重。

Doctor：**Have you ever smoked**?

医生：你抽烟么？

Patient：I stopped right after my first heart attack.

病人：第一次心脏病发作后我就不抽了。

Doctor：Quitting smoking is very challenging. It's so great that you stopped. **How much did you smoke**?

医生：戒烟很有难度。你能戒掉很好。你之前抽多少？

Patient：About two packs a day.

病人：大概一天两包。

Doctor：For how long?

医生：持续了多久？

Patient：Oh ... since I was 18.

病人：我想一下……从18岁开始。

Doctor：May I ask your age?

医生：我能问一下你的年龄么？

Patient：I'm 42.

病人：我 42 岁。

Doctor：**Have you ever had high blood pressure**?

医生：你有高血压么？

Patient：Yeah. My doctor gave me some medications for it，but I never asked for the refill after they ran out. I felt fine.

病人：是的。我的医生给了我一些药，但是我在药吃光后就没有再配了。我觉得我挺好的。

Doctor：Do you have diabetes?

医生：你有糖尿病么？

Patient：Thank goodness，I don't. My father does，though.

病人：还好我没有。但是我爸爸有。

Doctor：**Is there anyone else in your family who has diabetes**?

医生：你家里的其他人是否也患有糖尿病？

Patient：No.

病人：没有。

Doctor：Anyone else in your family who has had a heart attack?

医生：你家里其他人有没有心脏病？

Patient：I think my grandfather died of a heart attack.

病人：我觉得我外公就是死于心脏病发作。

Doctor：How old was he?

医生：他多大年纪？

Patient：At age 75.

病人：75 岁。

Doctor：What about your mother?

医生：你妈妈呢？

Patient：She died at age 64，right after my first heart attack. She had stomach cancer.

病人：她 64 岁的时候去世的，就在我第一次心脏病发作后。她有胃癌。

Doctor：Do you have any brothers or sisters?

医生：你有兄弟姐妹么?

Patient：My sister is 39 and she's fine.

病人：我妹妹 39 岁,她身体很好。

Doctor：Any other siblings?

医生：还有别的兄弟姐妹么?

Patient：My brother is 47. He had a heart attack when he was 38.

病人：我哥哥 47 岁。他在 38 岁时有过一次心脏病发作。

Doctor：Do you have any children?

医生：你有孩子么?

Patient：I have a boy who's 15.

病人：一个男孩,15 岁了。

Doctor：**How's your son's health**?

医生：你儿子健康情况怎么样?

Patient：No problem,but he's a little overweight.

病人：很好,除了有点超重。

Doctor：**Does anyone in your family have high blood pressure**? **Asthma**? **Tuberculosis**?

医生：你家中其他人是否患有高血压? 哮喘? 肺结核?

Patient：No.

病人：没有。

Doctor：**Have you ever been admitted here at our hospital**?

医生：你曾在我们医院住过院么?

Patient：No.

病人：没有。

Doctor：**Have you ever been hospitalized at any time other than for your heart attacks**?

医生：除了因为心脏病发作住院外,你有没有因为其他情况住院的?

Patient：I had my tonsil taken out when I was 16.

病人：我 16 岁的时候扁桃体摘除了。

Doctor：**Are you allergic to anything physically**?

医生：你对什么过敏么？

Patient：No.

病人：没有。

Doctor：**How was your health as a child**?

医生：你小时候健康情况怎么样？

Patient：Strong as a bull. I had the usual sore throats and ear aches that most kids get.

病人：身体很好。跟大多数孩子一样，有过常见的嗓子疼和耳朵痛。

Doctor：Did you have any of these illnesses? Chicken pox? Measles? Diphtheria? Polio? Mumps? Whooping cough? **Do you take any medications**?

医生：你患过这些疾病么？ 水痘、麻疹、白喉、小儿麻痹症、腮腺炎或百日咳或你有用过什么药么？

Patient：Just atenolol and isosorbide dinitrate.

病人：只有阿替洛尔和硝酸异山梨酯。

Doctor：Do you know the dosages?

医生：你知道剂量么？

Patient：I take 50 mg of atenolol once daily and 10 mg of isosorbide dinitrate 4 times a day.

病人：我每天服用一次 50 mg 阿替洛尔，硝酸异山梨酯 10 mg，一天 4 次。

Doctor：Do you think the medications ease the syndromes?

医生：你觉得药物能缓解症状么？

Patient：I guess so. I think I feel better with them.

病人：我觉得有。我觉得服药后好多了。

Doctor：Any other medications?

医生：还有别的药么？

Patient：Nitroglycerin ... when I get the pain.

病人：硝酸甘油，每当我感到疼的时候。

Doctor：Do you take any other medications? Over-the-counter medicines? Herbal medicines? Anything else?

医生：你还服用别的药物么？ 非处方药物、草药或其他？

Patient：I take Chlor-Trimeton when I catch a cold，but that's all about it.

病人：感冒时我会用氯苯那敏,仅此而已。

Doctor：**Have you ever had any other health problems**? Any problems with your liver? Kidneys? Stomach? Lungs? **How's your appetite**?

医生：你是否还有别的健康问题? 你的肝脏、肾脏、胃、肺都没有问题吧? 你的胃口怎么样?

Patient：No. Pretty good.

病人：没有。很好。

Doctor：Do you eat fish?

医生：你吃鱼么?

Patient：Sometimes.

病人：有时候。

Doctor：How often?

医生：频率呢?

Patient：Maybe ...Once every 3 weeks. I love shrimp, but I know it's not good for me.

病人：差不多每3周一次吧。我喜欢虾,但我知道这对我不好。

Doctor：**Have you had any weight fluctuations recently**?

医生：最近体重是否有变化?

Patient：I lost about 5 kg in the past 2 months.

病人：我在2个月内减重5公斤。

Doctor：Were you on a diet?

医生：你在减肥?

Patient：No, not exactly. I just haven't been too hungry lately.

病人：没有,我只是最近没有很饿。

Doctor：How's your sleep?

医生：你睡得怎么样?

Patient：Like a baby.

病人：像个孩子。

Doctor：I just have a few more questions for you. Do you drink alcohol?

医生：我还有一些问题。你喝酒么?

Patient：Occasionally, I suppose. Maybe after work, sometimes.

病人：我觉得也就是偶尔喝一下。有时会在下班后喝一点。

Doctor：**Have you ever felt the need to cut down on your drinking**?

医生：你觉得要减少酒精摄入么？

Patient：No.

病人：没有。

Doctor：**Have people annoyed you by criticizing your drinking**?

医生：其他人批评你喝酒时，你会觉得他们烦么？

Patient：Never, but my wife doesn't like me drinking.

病人：从来没有，但是我太太不喜欢我喝酒。

Doctor：**Have you ever felt bad or guilty about your drinking**?

医生：你会因为喝酒感到自责么？

Patient：Yeah. Once about 10 years ago my friend's father made some wine. We got really drunk ... it was terrible ... but never again!

病人：会的。10 年前有过一次，我朋友的爸爸酿了一些酒。我们喝得很醉，很糟糕，但是以后再不会发生了。

Doctor：Do you ever drive while intoxicated?

医生：你会酒后驾车么？

Patient：No! That's suicide.

病人：不！那是自杀。

Doctor：What's your typical day like?

医生：通常情况下，你的一天是怎么度过的？

Patient：Before I stopped working at the office, I got up about 5:30, dressed, and arrived at office by 7:30. I usually left the office about 7 and got home by 8:15. We'd have dinner, and I'd be in bed by 11:30, after the news.

病人：在我没停止工作前，我都是 5:30 起床，穿衣，7:30 到办公室。我通常晚上 7 点下班，8:15 到家。吃晚饭，我会在看完新闻后 11:30 上床睡觉。

Doctor：You can answer just "yes" or "no" to my following questions. Have you had any recent fevers?

医生：我接下来的问题，你可以回答"是"或"否"。最近有发烧么？

Patient：No.

病人：没有。

Doctor：Chills?

医生：寒战?

Patient：No.

病人：没有。

Doctor：Sweats?

医生：出汗?

Patient：No.

病人：没有。

Doctor：Rashes?

医生：出疹子?

Patient：No.

病人：没有。

Doctor：Changes in your hair or nails?

医生：头发或指甲有没有改变?

Patient：No.

病人：没有。

Doctor：Headaches?

医生：头痛?

Patient：Rarely, about once every 2 to 3 months.

病人：很少,大致每2—3个月有一次吧。

Doctor：**For how long have you been having headaches**?

医生：头痛症状出现多久了?

Patient：Years. ... I guess about 15 to 20 years.

病人：有年头了。我想大概是15—20年。

Doctor：Can you tell me something about your headache?

医生：你能描述一下你的头疼情况么?

Patient：They're right here and feels like stabbing pain. They last about 1 to 2 hours.

病人：就在这,而且是一种刺痛。持续1—2小时。

Doctor：What relieves them?

医生：有什么缓解办法么?

Patient：Usually aspirin.

病人：通常是服用阿司匹林。

Doctor：**Have you noticed a change in the pattern or severity of your headaches**?

医生：你有没有注意到头痛规律或严重程度的改变？

Patient：No.

病人：没有。

Doctor：Have you had any head injuries?

医生：你有过头部创伤么？

Patient：Never.

病人：从来没有。

Doctor：Have you ever fainted?

医生：你有昏厥过么？

Patient：No.

病人：没有。

Useful Structures

1. What seems to be the problem?

   您遇到了什么问题？

2. How did you feel when you were discharged from the hospital?

   出院时感觉怎么样？

3. Have you ever smoked?

   你抽烟么？

4. How much did you smoke?

   你之前抽多少？

5. Have you ever had high blood pressure?

   你有高血压么？

6. Is there anyone else in your family who has diabetes?

   你家里的其他人是否也患有糖尿病？

7. How's your son's health?

   你儿子健康情况怎么样？

8. Have you ever been admitted here at our hospital?

   你曾在我们医院住过院么？

9. Have you ever been hospitalized at any time other than for your heart attacks?

   除了因为心脏病发作住院外,你有没有因为其他情况住院的？

10. Have you ever been hospitalized for any other conditions?

    你有因为其他原因住院么？

11. Are you allergic to anything physically?

    你有对什么过敏么？

12. How was your health as a child?

    你小时候健康情况怎么样？

13. Do you take any medications?

    你有用过什么药么？

14. Have you ever had any other health problems?

    你是否还有别的健康问题？

15. How's your appetite?

    你的胃口怎么样？

16. Have you had any weight fluctuations/change recently?

    最近体重是否有变化？

17. Have you ever felt the need to cut down on your drinking?

    你觉得要减少酒精摄入么？

18. Have people annoyed you by criticizing your drinking?

    其他人批评你喝酒时,你会觉得他们烦么？

19. Have you ever felt bad or guilty about your drinking?

    你会因为喝酒感到自责么？

20. For how long have you been having headaches?

    头痛症状出现多久了？

21. Have you noticed a change in the pattern or severity of your headaches?

    你有没有注意到头痛规律或严重程度的改变？

Part Three

Exercises

• Put the following expressions from Chinese into English.

1. 病历_____
2. 病史来源_____
3. 病史可信度_____
4. 职业史_____
5. 环境史_____
6. 健康维持_____
7. 物质滥用_____
8. 当前用药_____

9. Chief complaint is characterized as the one or more _____（症状）or concerns causing the patient to _____（医疗照护）.

10. _____（现有疾病）includes patient's _____（想法）and _____（感受）about the illness, may include _____（药物）, _____ _____（过敏）, and tobacco use and _____（酒精）, which are frequently _____（相关）the _____（现有疾病）.

11. _____（既往病史）lists _____（儿童期）and _____（成年期）illnesses, includes _____（健康维持）practices such as _____（免疫接种）, _____（筛查测试）, _____ _____（生活方式）, and home safety.

12. _____（家族史）outlines age and health, or age and _____ _____（死亡原因）, of _____（兄妹）, parents, and grandparents, documents presence or absence of specific illnesses in family, such as _____（高血压）, _____（糖尿病）, or type of cancer.

13. _____（个人和社会史）describes educational level, _____（原生家庭）, current household, _____（个人兴趣）and lifestyle.

• Fill in the blanks to complete the written history of Mr. Smith according to the dialogue in Part Two.

Chief Complaint： _____ for the past 6 months.

History of Current Illness: This is the first Nanjing First Hospital _____ for Mr. Smith, a 42-year-old lawyer with coronary artery disease. He suffered his first _____ in 2012. He was _____ for 2 weeks in XX hospital. Six months later, he _____ from his second heart attack. He was again _____ at XX hospital. He was started on some _____ for his condition. Over the past 6 months, the patient has had increasing chest pain with _____ down his _____.

The patient's chest pain is _____ by exercise and emotion. The patient takes _____ as needed, with relief within 5 minutes. The patient's _____ for coronary artery disease include a history of untreated _____, a 40 _____ history of smoking (2 packs per day for 20 years), and a brother with a _____ at the age of 38 years. The patient denies any history of _____.

Past Medical History: The patient was _____ at age 16 years for an _____. The only other hospitalizations were for the patient's two heart attacks, as indicated previously. His only medications are indicated in the history of current illness. There is no history of _____, _____, _____ or _____ disease. There is no history of _____.

Family History: The patient's father has a history of _____. The patient's mother died at age 64 years from _____. The patient's older brother, as mentioned previously, is 47 years of age and has _____. The patient has a younger sister who is 39 years of age and is well. There is no history of _____. The patient is married and has a 15-year-old son, who is well.

Part Four

Other Structures

Past Medical History 病史

1. How has your health been in the past?

   你过去的健康状况怎么样？

2. Have you ever been involved in a serious accident?

你有没有遭受过严重的意外?

3. Have you ever been in therapy or counseling?

你参加过治疗或咨询么?

4. What emotional problems have you had?

你有过什么情绪问题?

5. Have you ever been hospitalized for a nonmedical or nonsurgical reason?

你是否曾因为非医疗或非手术原因住院?

6. How do you know you are allergic?

你是怎么知道自己过敏的?

7. What kind of problem did you have when you took ... ?

你在服用/吃……的时候,出现了什么样的问题?

8. Do you use nicotine in any form: cigarettes, cigars, pipes, chewing tobacco?

你有吸食任何形式的尼古丁么:香烟、雪茄、烟管、咀嚼用烟草?

9. Please tell me about your drinking of alcohol.

请告诉我你的酒精摄入情况。

10. Have you ever used drugs other than those required for medical reasons?

除了医学治疗用途的药物,你有用过别的药物么?

11. Do you use drugs other than those prescribed by a physician?

你是否用过不是由医师开具的处方药?

12. Has your diet changed recently?

你的饮食最近发生什么变化了么?

13. What kinds of foods do you like or dislike, why?

你喜欢或不喜欢吃什么,为什么?

14. Do you have any food intolerance?

你有食物不耐受么?

15. Do you have trouble falling asleep?

你有入睡困难么?

16. Do you stay asleep the whole night, or do you awaken in the middle of the night, unable to go back to sleep?

你能睡整晚么,还是说半夜会醒过来,然后就不能入睡了?

17. Many patients frequently use other kinds of therapy when they have the

symptoms you described. Have you used or thought about using massage, herbs, acupuncture, vitamin or other different therapies?

许多病人在有你描述的这些症状时,他们通常会使用别的治疗方法。你有没有使用过或考虑过使用推拿、草药、针灸、维生素或其他治疗方法?

Occupational and Environmental History 既往病史

1. What type of work do you do?
   你从事何种工作?

2. How long have you been doing this work?
   你做这个工作有多久了?

3. Are you exposed to any hazardous materials? Do you ever use protective equipment?
   你有没有暴露在任何有害物质下? 你有用过防护性设备么?

4. What kind of work did you do before you had your current job?
   在这份工作之前,你从事的是何种工作?

5. Where do you live? For how long?
   你住在哪里? 住了多久?

6. Have you ever lived near any factories, shipyards, or other potentially hazardous facilities?
   你之前是否住在工厂、船厂或其他潜在危险场所的附近?

7. Do you now have, or have you previously had, environmental or occupational exposures to asbestos, lead, fumes, chemicals, dusts, loud noise, radiation, or other toxic factors?
   你是否知道你现在,或你以前有过环境或职业暴露,如石棉、铅、废气、化学物质、灰尘、噪音、辐射或其他毒性物质?

Family History 家族病史

- Are you aware of any genetically determined disease in the family?
  你有注意到家族中有任何基因型疾病么?

Summary 总结

1. Is there anything else you would like to tell me that I have not already asked?

   有其他我没问，但你想补充的么？

2. Are there any questions you might like to ask?

   你有什么问题想问么？

Part Five

Supplementary Reading: What Is My Medical History?

When you fill out forms at your doctor's office, do you wonder why it matters whether or not your grandmother had high blood pressure or diabetes? Your doctor also asks you questions like this. Why is it important?

Your medical history includes both your personal health history and your family health history. Your personal health history has details about any health problems you've ever had. A family health history has details about health problems your blood relatives have had during their lifetimes.

This information gives your doctor all kinds of important clues about what's going on with your health, because many diseases run in families. The history also tells your doctor what health issues you may be at risk for in the future. If your doctor learns, for example, that both of your parents have heart disease, he may focus on your heart health when you're much younger than other patients who don't have a family history of heart disease.

Who to Include

If it's possible, every adult should know their family health history. You may or may not already know some information about conditions that affected different family members. Even if you think you do, double-check what you know. Find out even more about as many blood relatives as you can, and remember to include half-sisters and brothers.

You should not include people who are not blood relatives, such as:

- Your spouse
- Your adopted children or adoptive parents/siblings
- Your step children or step-siblings
- Your relatives who married into the family

Gather Your Family Health History

Make sure to write down what you learn, in case you forget details over time. You'll also be able to add to the information you already have.

Make sure to share the information with your siblings, children, or grandchildren, as they get older.

To get started, call your relatives, or ask them in person about your family health history. Let your relatives know you're not being nosy, but just want to gather details that could keep you and other family members healthy. You can offer to share what you learn, so that everyone can benefit from your research.

You'll want to ask about common chronic (ongoing) health conditions. Find out how old each person was when they learned about their condition. You may want to start by asking about these common family health problems:

- Cancer
- Heart disease
- Diabetes
- High blood pressure
- High cholesterol
- Stroke

You'll need to know the health history of relatives who have died, too. If you have access to death certificates or medical records, you can find out the cause of death and how old they were, but living relatives may know the details.

If You're Adopted

If you were adopted, you may not know anything about your birth parents' health history. If that's the case, a big chunk of your medical history is a question mark. You may wonder if you're at risk for heart disease, cancer, or other diseases that run in families.

Rules vary by state, but most adopted people are able to access details about their birth parents' family medical history once they become adults. Such information may be found through the department that assists with adoptions.

How Your History Keeps You Healthy

Once you find out your medical history, you can make powerful choices for yourself. If you learn, for example, that heart disease runs in your family, you may decide to make lifestyle changes that could lower your risk, such as quitting smoking, losing weight, or getting more exercise.

Your doctor may also use the information to give you screening tests, which might catch a disease, such as like cancer, early. There are lots of ways your medical history can put you and your doctor in better control of your health.

Part Six

Conversational English Functions

- Agreement and Disagreement 同意与不同意

1. Asking If someone Agrees

Don't you agree with me?

Don't you think so?

You'd agree with me, wouldn't you?

All right with you?

Do you go along with that?

Can I ask you if you would agree that ... ?

Right?

2. Agreeing

I absolutely/totally/entirely agree.

I can't help thinking the same.

I couldn't agree more.

I think you are right.

You know, that's exactly what I think.

That's a good point/idea.

I take your point.

That's right/true.

I suppose so.

Oh, exactly/definitely/absolutely.

I'm with you on that.

I'd go along with you on that/there.

3. Disagreeing

I disagree.

Do you really think so?

I can't accept that.

I wouldn't go along with you there/on that.

I don't think so.

I'm afraid you're quite wrong.

I'm not sure if I would agree with you on that.

I see things rather differently myself.

I'm afraid I can't accept your argument.

I'm not at all convinced by your explanation.

You can't be serious!

Come off it!

You must be joking!

Don't be silly!

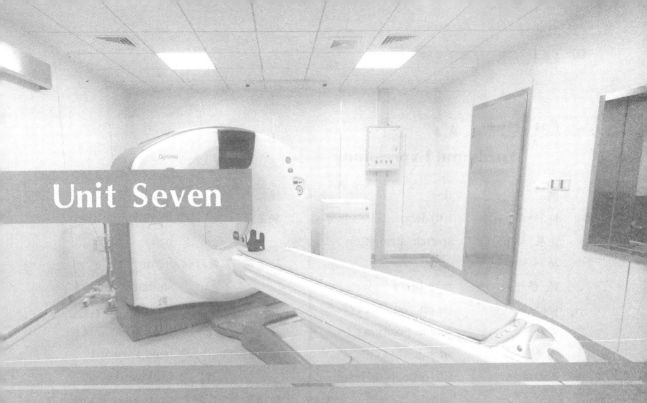

Unit Seven

Physical Examinations
身体检查

Learning Objectives

熟悉与身体部位及身体检查相关的词汇及表达

掌握与身体检查相关的句型结构

掌握礼貌用语的表达

了解中英文礼貌用语表达方式的异同

Outline

✓音、视频资源

✓参考答案

✓学术探讨

Part One

Words and Expressions

躺	lie	摸	touch
仰/倾斜	tilt/drop	躺床上	lie down on the bed
伸展/伸直	stretch/straighten		
动一下	move	趴着躺下/俯卧位	lie on your stomach/prone position
脱/移开	take off/remove		
仰卧位	lie on your back/ supine position	屈膝	bend your knees
侧坐	sit sideways	向前/后倾	bend forward/ backward
头部后仰	tilt/drop your head back	按压腹部	press your stomach
量体温	take one's temperature	将头转向右边	turn your head to the right side
抬起小腿	lift your leg up/ raise your leg	卷起衣袖	pull/curl/roll up your sleeves
脱下鞋子	take off your shoes		

Part Two

Model Dialogues

Stomachache 腹痛

Doctor: You are looking very pale. **I would like to take your temperature**. Can you put this under your arm/oxter?

医生:你看起来脸色不好,我要给你量下体温。把这个放在腋下,好吗?

Patient: Yes, sure.

病人:好的。

Doctor: **I need to examine you. Could you just lie down on the bed** and pull up your coat and loosen your trousers.

医生：我现在要给你做检查。请躺在床上。把衣服卷起来、裤带松开。

Patient：OK.

病人：好的。

Doctor：**Please show me where it hurts**.

医生：请指给我看哪里疼吧。

Patient：Just there.

病人：就那里。

Doctor：**Take it easy**. I'm going to press your stomach and **please tell me if it hurts.**

医生：放轻松。我要按压你的肚子，疼的话告诉我。

Patient：Just there. When you pressed it, it hurts.

病人：就是那里，你一按就痛。

Doctor：**Would you mind turning to your left side for me**? Tell me if you feel any pain when I press here.

医生：你能左侧卧吗？我按这里的时候你觉得疼也告诉我。

Patient：No, I don't have any pain there.

病人：那里不疼。

Doctor：OK, I've finished now. Please get dressed and sit here.

医生：好的。我检查完了。穿好坐这来。

Useful Structures

1. I would like to（take your temperature）.

   我将要（给你量体温）

2. Could you just（lie down on your bed）?

   你可以（躺在床上）吗？

3. I need to examine you.

   我需要给你做个检查。

4. Take it easy.

   放轻松。

5. Please show me where it hurts.

请告诉我哪里疼。

6. Please tell me if it hurts.

如果痛就告诉我。

7. Would you mind (turning to your left side for me)?

您介意(左侧卧)吗?

Part Three

Exercises

- Put the following sentences into English.

1. 我要量下血压。

_____

2. 伸直左腿。

_____

3. 卷起袖子。

_____

4. 仰卧,头转向侧边。

_____

5. 右侧卧躺着。

_____

6. 请您躺着别动。

_____

7. 我能动一下你的拇指吗?

_____

8. 如果不舒服请您告诉我。

_____

9. 我需要听下你的肺部，请把外套解开，坐靠近点。

_____

_____

10. 请您侧对着我坐，头尽量别动，我要检查一下您的耳朵。谢谢配合。

_____

_____

• **Put the following dialogues from English into Chinese.**

1. Doctor: Would you slip off your top things, please. Now I just want to see you standing. Hands by your side. You're sticking that hip out a little bit, aren't you?

Patient: Yes, well. I can't straighten up easily.

Doctor: Could you bend down as far as you can with your knees straightening and stop when you've had enough.

Patient: That's the limit.

Doctor: Not very far, is it? Stand up again. Now I would like you to lean backwards. All right. That's not much either. Now stand up straight again.

2. Doctor: Now first of all, I would like you to slide your right hand down the right side of your thigh. See how far you can go. That's fine. Now do the same thing on the opposite side. Fine. Now just come back to standing straight. Now keep your feet together just as they are. Keep your knees firm. Now try and turn both shoulders round to the right. Look right round. Keep your knees and feet steady.

Patient: Oh, that's sore.

Doctor: Go back to the center again. Now try the same thing and go round to the left side. Fine. Now back to the center. That's fine. Now would you like to get onto the couch and lie on your face? I'm just going to try and find out where the sore spot is.

• Fill in the blanks according to the picture to complete the following instructions about physical examinations.

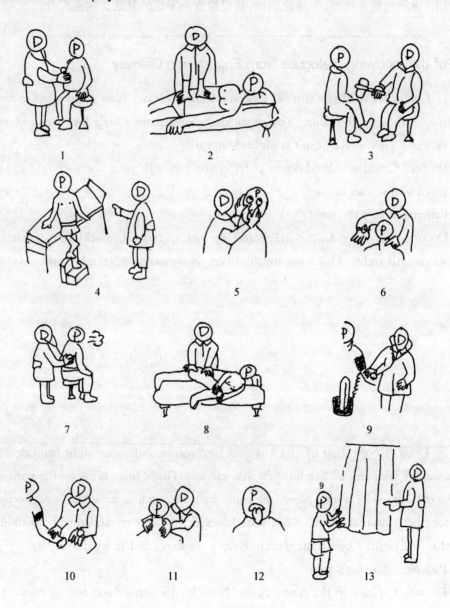

1

2

3

4

5

6

7

8

9

10

11

12

13

1. Right, now I want to listen to your heart. Just _____ _____ quietly.

2. I would like to feel your abdomen. Put your arms down _____ your side and let your _____ relax. That is it. Are there any places tender or _____? Now I want to check your liver and spleen. So take a deep breath in and hold it ... fine ...

3. Let me check the _____ in your arms and legs with the little hammer. Relax! Try not to tighten up.

4. Hop on the table for me, are you _____ of doing it by yourself? Shall I give you a _____?

5. Now let's have a look _____ your _____. Look _____ for me please.

6. _____ your head to the _____ to look at the wall; I will check the pulse in your _____.

7. Now sit forward when I listen to your back, hold breath ... Good. Now let's listen to your lungs. Take deep _____ through your mouth in ... and _____ ... keep going.

8. I'd just like to examine your prostate and rectum. Now this will be slightly _____, but it wouldn't _____. Lie down on your _____ _____ and _____ your knees right up to your chest. Fine. I am going to _____ a finger into your rectum. Don't worry, you won't _____ any control.

9. Now let's take your _____ _____. _____ your arm, please.

10. Right, give me a _____, will you? I am going to _____ your _____. That is fine.

11. Let me feel your _____ pipe. Let me just _____ your glands. That is fine.

12. _____ _____ your tongue for me please. _____ your mouth and say "Ah".

13. Now Mr. Jacob, I'd like to _____ you. I just want to check one or two things, your heart, your _____ and _____. Would you just take off your clothes down to your underwear? Put on this _____ with the opening on its back.

Part Four

Other Structures

1. You might feel a little bit of discomfort.

    你可能会觉得有些不舒服。

2. It won't take long.

    时间不会长。

3. It will tickle a bit but won't be sore.

    可能会有些痒，但不疼。

4. Please lie down on your back.

    请平躺着。

5. Please breathe normally/slowly.

    请正常/慢慢呼吸。

6. Take a deep breath please.

    请深呼吸。

7. Hold your breath and follow my instructions.

    屏住呼吸听我指令。

8. Please relax the muscles of your abdomen/stomach and show me where the trouble/discomfort is.

    请把腹部肌肉放松。指给我看哪儿不舒服。

9. Please turn around and show me your back.

    请转过来让我看看你的背。

10. Please lift your arms to the side.

    请把手臂水平侧向伸出。

11. Please put your arms forward.

    请把手臂前伸。

12. Please touch the back of your head with left hand.

    请用左手碰你的后脑勺。

13. Please raise your right / left arm as high as you can.

    请将右臂/左臂尽量抬高。

14. Can you touch your shoulder blade with your right/left hand?

你能用右手/左手摸着你的肩胛骨吗?

15. Please sit down and face me and drop your head back.

请您面向我坐好,头向后仰。

16. Please relax and try not to blink.

请放松,尽量不要眨眼。

17. Now I will examine your throat, please open your mouth wide and say "Ah".

现在我要检查一些你的咽喉,请张开嘴说"啊"。

Part Five

Supplementary Reading: Polite Words and Phrases

Have you ever been around someone who motivates you to become a better person? Typically, that person is polite in all areas, including the way he or she speaks. Someone who doesn't employ a speech filter but needs to probably doesn't have your respect.

Some folks might consider using polite language an outdated etiquette rule, but it isn't. There are plenty of people whose respect you want, so why risk offending them?

Even people who are polite in every other way may have a bad habit of using rude language. You can't do anything about other people's bad manners, but you can work on your own.

Don't expect overnight success if you have a bad habit of letting bad language fly. It takes time, but it's worth it.

Polite Phrases

Most people learn the importance of the magic words "please" and "thank you" at a very early age. As you go through life, you see that better things happen when you don't forget to say them.

Not only do people warm up to you more quickly but they also want to be around you more and for longer periods of time. In fact, although they may not tell you, they might even consider you their role model.

Foul Language

Foul language has been around forever, but it has never been more widely used than it is now. What's sad is that it shows a lack of respect for people who don't speak that way.

Many older people find it offensive, and most parents don't want their children cursing or using words that were once considered socially unacceptable. Finding another way to express yourself will put you in good graces with these people.

Language Etiquette

Proper etiquette goes way beyond how to set a table for a formal dinner and proper use of utensils. It's even more than knowing how to shake hands with someone you've just met. Good manners should be incorporated into every aspect of your life, including what you say during the most informal of times.

Pet Peeves

An occasional slip-up happens to most people. So if you make a mistake and say something you shouldn't, apologize and move on. The folks around you probably won't remember unless you make a big deal of your faux pas, so don't dwell on it.

Foul language isn't the only thing people use inappropriately. For example, someone might be in the habit of grunting instead of responding to another person's greeting.

Also, if you have formed habits such as saying, "No problem," after being thanked, you might want to rethink that because those words don't make sense in the context of the conversation. When someone says, "Thank you," she's not stating a problem. "You're welcome," is much more appropriate.

Never Too Late

Even if you haven't used these polite words and phrases all your life, it's never too late to start. Practice holding polite conversations with family and close friends until you're comfortable and it feels natural. Eventually, speaking politely will become second nature to you.

Common Polite Words and Phrases

Here are some of the most common words and phrases that anyone who cares about proper etiquette should incorporate into their everyday language:

Please—This is one of those words that can show good manners or come across as sarcastic, based on your tone. Any time you ask for something, it's always a good idea to add this word to soften the request. Use it in a way that shows your sincerity.

You're welcome—When someone says, "Thank you," your instant response should be, "You're welcome," "You're certainly welcome," or some variation that feels comfortable to you. Another way to express the same thought is, "I was happy to do it," or, "My pleasure."

Thank you—When someone does something nice for you or gives you a gift, you should always say, "Thank you," even if it's not something you like. Not doing so gives the impression that you feel entitled to whatever it is, and that can leave a sour taste in a mannerly person's mouth.

May I—The phrase "may I" puts you on the same side as the person you are speaking to, and you sound less demanding than if you were to leave it out. It gives the other person the feeling that you empathize, without you having to say that. For example, when you say, "May I see that book?" you give the person an opportunity to share what she is looking at.

Excuse me—This is an acknowledgement that you are asking forgiveness for leaving the table, coughing, or otherwise disrupting something you are engaged in.

Pardon me—This phrase is interchangeable with "excuse me." Pardon me sounds more formal.

I beg your pardon—Some people, would say "What?" when asking someone to repeat what they'd just said. Many of us were told that "I beg your pardon" was much more polite and less harsh. The origin of this phrase was used to release someone from punishment.

I'm sorry—When you make a mistake, hurt someone's feelings, or do something that you know you shouldn't have done, saying, "I'm sorry," is always the first thing you should say. You're acknowledging your faux pas and letting the other person know you regret having done whatever it was.

Words and phrases that need to be eradicated from your vocabulary:

No problem—When someone is thanked, and that person in turn says, "No problem," some people cringe. Even though it's the contemporary way of saying, "You're welcome," it seems abrupt and can be confusing to anyone who grew up without that expression.

Yep, yeah, and nope—These words are rude versions of "yes" and "no." The proper words are only one syllable and just as easy to say, so why not simply use them?

Any curse words—Curse words might have been used originally for shock value, but when they become part of your everyday language, they stop shocking people. They also make you sound crude and may offend people who don't use them. It's best not to use any words you wouldn't want your mom or grandmother to hear. If you're around anyone who uses those words, calling them out will probably have no effect. Maybe you can set an example for how to speak politely.

Any words that are sexist, racist, or derogatory to a specific group. Derogatory language shows a lack of respect for others, and there is never an appropriate time to use it. If using these terms has become a habit, do everything in your power to break it because it is offensive and can get you into serious trouble.

Polite language is always appropriate, so why not use it? Speaking to others with respect won't offend others, and it just might actually win a few friends and help you get ahead in business.

Part Six

Conversational English Functions

- Asking for Information 询问信息

1. Asking for Information

Can you tell me something about it?

I hope you don't mind my asking, but I'd like to know ...

I should be interested to know the fact.

I wonder whether you could help me. I'd like to know ...

I wonder if you could explain about it in more detail.

Could you tell me some more about it?

Excuse me, do you know how to ... ?

Something else I'd like to know is ...

Would you mind telling me ... ?

2. Asking If Somebody Knows Something

Have you got some idea about ... ?

Are you aware of ... ?

Can you give me any information about ... , please?

I wonder whether you could let me know something about ...

Has anybody told you that ... ?

You know about ... , don't you?

Did you happen to know anything about ... ?

You know that, don't you?

3. Expressing Knowledge of Something

I've been told about ...

Somebody has told me about that.

Yes, I do know ...

That's what I heard.

For all I know, ...

I am fully aware of that.

I am quite aware that ...

My information is that ...

4. Expressing Ignorance of Something

I'm afraid I don't know much about it.

I'm afraid I've no idea ...

I'm quite in the dark about it.

I'm sorry I haven't got the faintest/slightest idea.

That's news to me.

I haven't got a clue about ...

I couldn't tell ...

5. Additional Information

Would/Could/Can you tell me more about ... ?

Do you know anything else?

Sorry to press you, but could you tell me ... ?

Sorry, I don't quite understand. Could you tell me ... ?

And one more question ...

I'd like to know some more about ...

6. Checking If You Have Been Understood

Am I making myself clear?

Did I make everything clear?

Do you know/see what I mean?

Do you understand what I said?

Are you following me (so far)?

Have you got all that?

Do you think you've got it?

Do you see my point?

Does that seem to make sense?

Is that clear to you?

Didn't you see the point?

You got it, didn't you?

Are you with me (so far)?

Know what I'm getting at?

OK so far?

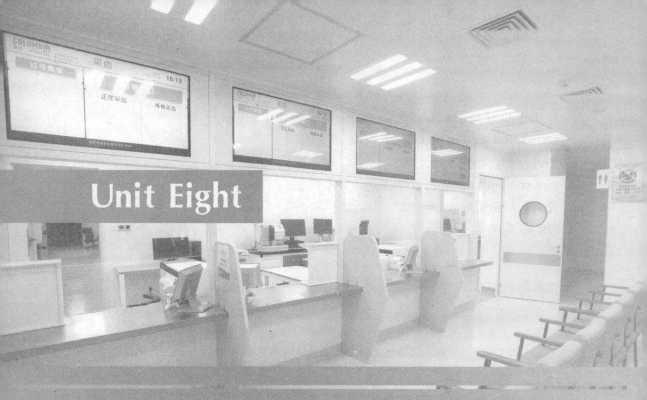

Unit Eight

Examinations，Tests and Diagnoses
检查、化验及诊断

Learning Objectives

> 熟悉各类检查化验的英文说法
>
> 掌握与检查、化验及诊断相关的句型结构

Outline

✓音、视频资源

✓参考答案

✓学术探讨

Part One

Words and Expressions

化验	test	报告单	report
化验单	test form	样本瓶	specimen bottle/pot
化验结果	test result	尿液	urine
化验室	laboratory	粪便样本	stool specimen
容器	container	尿常规检查	urine routine
粪便	stool	培养	culture
粪便化验	stool test	血液检查	blood test
尿液分析	urinalysis	抽血	blood draw
敏感度	sensitivity	末梢采血	finger stick/finger prick
血糖检查	blood glucose test		
静脉穿刺采血	venipuncture	钡餐	barium meal
肾功能检查	renal function	关节造影	arthrography/ radiography of the joint
造影	radiography		
X 光	X-ray		
B 超	Ultrasound B/B-Mode Ultrasound	腹部 X 光检查	X-ray of stomach
		胸部 B 超检查	Ultrasound B of the chest
脑 CT 检查	CT scan of the brain		
核磁共振	MRI (Magnetic Resonance Imaging)	（增强）CT	(enhanced) CT scan
		心电图检查	ECG(electrocardiogram) test
输血	blood transfusion		
（无痛）胃镜	(painless) gastroscopy	静脉注射	IV drip
		（无痛）肠镜	(painless) colonoscopy

Part Two
Model Dialogues

Headache 头痛

Doctor：I need to check your eyes, please bend forward slightly and look straight ahead for me.

医生：我现在要检查你的眼睛,请略微弯下腰直视我。

Patient：The light is very painful.

病人：光照着疼。

Doctor：Yes, your headache causes photophobia on you.

医生：是的,你的头痛导致你畏光。

Doctor：**You need to have a blood test, and here is the form,** and the nurse will show you where to go.

医生：你需要验血,这是化验单,护士会带你去。

Patient：Do I need to come back tomorrow?

病人：我明天还需要来吗?

Doctor：No. **Please wait for the results and bring them back to me. It will take about 30 minutes.**

医生：不用,你等化验结果出来直接拿给我,大概30分钟就好。

30 minutes later 30分钟过后

Doctor：**The test shows nothing unusual, but you may have got a bad migraine.** If it gets worse, you will need to have a CT or MRI scan.

医生：你的化验结果表明没有什么特别问题,应该是偏头痛。如果越来越严重,可能需要做CT或者核磁共振检查。

Urinary Infection 尿路感染

Doctor：May I examine you please?

医生：我能给你做个身体检查吗?

Patient：Yes, please doctor.

病人：可以的，医生。

Doctor：Please take off your coat, lie on the bed. You can cover yourself with the blanket.

医生：请脱掉外套躺在床上。你可以盖上毯子。

Patient：Sure.

病人：好的。

After the examination 检查过后

Doctor：**It seems you have an acute urinary tract infection. We need to test the function of your kidney.** I think **you need to have the urine routine, some blood tests** and an ultrasound B of your kidney. I'll also send your urine specimen for urinalysis, culture and sensitivity. Here are the forms.

医生：你可能尿路感染了。我们要查一下你的肾脏功能。你需要做尿常规检查、血液检查和肾脏 B 超。还要把你的尿液样本送去做尿液分析、尿培养和药敏试验。这是化验单。

Patient：Where can I get the bottle for the urine specimen?

病人：请问哪里拿样本瓶?

Doctor：Over there.

医生：在那里。

Patient：Could I have/take the tests now?

病人：我现在就可以去化验检查吗?

Doctor：Yes. **Please come to me again with the test results.**

医生：是的。化验结果出来后复诊。

After the tests 化验过后

Doctor：Show me the report please.

医生：请给我看下检查报告。

Patient：Here you are.

病人：给您。

Doctor：**The tests show that you have a problem with your kidney. It's called acute pyelonephritis.**

医生：化验结果显示你肾脏出了些问题。这种病叫急性肾盂肾炎。

Patient：**Do I need to be hospitalized**?

病人：我需要住院治疗吗？

Doctor：No. If the symptoms get worse，come to the Emergency Department immediately.

医生：不需要。如果病情恶化马上来急诊。

Useful Structures

1. You need to have (a blood test).

    你需要去(验血)。

2. You need to have an ultrasound of (your kidney).

    您需要做(肾脏)B超。

3. Here is the form.

    这是化验单。

4. Please wait for the results and bring them back to me.

    请等待结果然后带给我。

5. Please come to me again with the test results.

    化验结果出来后复诊。

6. It will take about 30 minutes.

    大概需要30分钟。

7. Show me the report please.

    请给我看下检查报告。

8. It seems you have/may have(an acute urinary tract infection).

    您可能(尿路感染了)。

9. We need to test the function of your kidney.

    我们需要检查一下您的肾功能。

10. The test shows nothing unusual/that you have a problem with (your kidney).

    检查结果表明没有什么异常/你的(肾脏)有些问题。

11. It's called "acute pyelonephritis".

    这种病叫作急性肾盂肾炎。

12. Do I need to be hospitalized/admitted to hospital?

我需要住院治疗吗?

Part Three

Exercises

• Put the following sentences into English.

1. 我需要你的粪便样本。

_____

2. 我需要测一下您的血糖。

_____

3. 你需要拍一下胸部超声波扫描。

_____

4. 这是样本瓶。

_____

5. 这是 X 光片图。

_____

6. 请把您的尿液样本带到化验室等待化验结果。

_____

7. 我们需要检查您的肝功能。

_____

8. 请等待大约一小时,化验结果出来后复诊。

_____

9. 化验结果正常。

_____

10. 您可能得了麻疹(measles)。

_____

11. 检查结果表明您的胃有点问题。这种病叫胃溃疡。

_____

12. 化验结果表明你需要静脉注射。

• Make a dialogue about "chest pain" with the model dialogues in Unit 7 and Unit 8 as the reference.

The possible contents include: physical examination, tests recommendation, results and diagnosis (pulmonary embolism). You can begin with "There is a blood clot in your left leg ..."

Part Four

Other Structures

1. I will tell you where the bacteriology department is.
   我会告诉你细菌室在哪里。

2. Please bring it back to the Bacteriology Department. I will tell you where to go.
   请将装了尿液的瓶子带回细菌室。我会告诉你怎么过去。

3. Please take the specimen there and wait for the results.
   请带着样本过去,然后等候结果。

4. Please pay for the tests. The report will be given shortly.
   请将化验单缴费,报告很快就会出来。

5. You need to fill up to a third of this container.
   你需要装到这个容器的三分之一。

6. Please empty your bladder.
   请排空尿液。

7. How long have you been fasting/been on an empty stomach?
   您空腹多久了?

8. I need a mid-stream/24-hour specimen of urine.
   我需要您小便中段/24 小时的尿液样本。

9. You don't need to collect the first or last part of urine that comes out. Collect the mid-stream urine in a container.

你不需要收集前段和后段尿。用容器收集中段尿。

10. Here is a bottle to collect it in.

    这是收集瓶。

11. Please use a clean jug or container to collect your urine, and then pour into the bottle.

    请用干净的壶或容器收集你的尿液,然后倒入到收集瓶里。

12. Please wait in the waiting area for 30 minutes. Do not hesitate to tell me if you feel uncomfortable.

    请在等待室等待30分钟。如果不舒服请立刻告诉我。

13. You will need to collect the results in ... days.

    ……天后结果就能出来。

14. You will have to go to the X-ray Department, please take this form.

    你需要去放射室,请带着这张化验单。

15. You will need to have a full bladder before the ultrasound.

    在做超声波扫描前,请憋尿,使膀胱充盈。

16. Please drink ... glasses of water before you have the scan.

    请在做超声波扫描前喝……杯水。

17. Please drink plenty of water in 24 hours to speed up the excretion of contrast agent.

    请24小时内喝大量的水以加速造影剂的排泄。

18. You need to have an empty stomach.

    您需要空腹。

19. I'm putting some cream/gel on your wrists and ankles.

    我将在您手腕和脚踝处涂上一些凝胶。

20. Now I'm going to swab your back. You'll feel a bit cold.

    我要擦拭您的后背。您会觉得有些凉。

21. Try to keep still as possibly as you can.

    尽量保持不动。

22. Please lay your arm on the table ... clench your fist ... unleash it.

    请把手臂平放在桌上……握拳……松开。

23. Please keep the gauze on for at least 15 minutes.

　　　请将纱布保留至少 15 分钟。

24. Please press the cotton pad for 5 to 10 minutes until there is no bleeding.

　　　请按压棉球 5—10 分钟,一直到没有血液渗出。

25. Please keep your report bar code.

　　　请保管好您取报告的条形码。

26. Take the report bar code to the self-service machine to print the report.

　　　请将报告条形码拿到自助机上打印报告。

27. Your pulse is a bit irregular. I think we'll have to get a tracing of your heartbeat.

　　　您的心跳有些不正常。我们需要继续跟踪您的心跳。

28. It's possible that you have a condition called (glaucoma) which is caused by (increased pressure inside the eye).

　　　您可能患上了(青光眼),这种疾病是由(眼压升高)引起的。

29. Your MRI scan confirms that you've got (a damaged disc in the lower part of your back).

　　　您的核磁共振检查确认您(腰椎间盘有损伤)。

Part Five

Supplementary Reading: What to Know about COVID-19 Diagnosis

The outbreak of the new coronavirus disease, which was first outbroken in China in December 2019, is continuing to affect people across the globe.

Early and accurate diagnosis of COVID-19—the disease caused by an infection with the new coronavirus—is critical to curbing its spread and improving health outcomes.

Keep reading to find out what to do if you think you have symptoms of COVID-19, and which tests are currently being used to diagnose this disease in the United States.

When to consider getting tested for a COVID-19 diagnosis

If you've been exposed to the virus or show mild symptoms of COVID-19, call your doctor for advice about how and when to get tested. Don't go to your doctor's office in person, as you could be contagious.

You can also access the Centers for Disease Control and Prevention's (CDC) to help you decide when to get tested or seek medical care.

<u>**Symptoms to watch out for**</u>

The most common symptoms reported by people with COVID-19 include:

- fever
- cough
- fatigue
- shortness of breath

Some people may have other symptoms, too, such as:

- a sore throat
- headache
- runny or stuffy nose
- diarrhea
- muscle aches and pains
- chills
- repeated shaking with chills
- loss of smell or taste

The symptoms of COVID-19 typically appear within 2 to 14 days after initial exposure to the virus.

Some people show few to no signs of illness during the early phase of infection but can still transmit the virus to others.

In mild cases, home care and self-quarantine measures may be all that is needed to fully recover and keep the virus from spreading to others. But some cases call for more complex medical interventions.

<u>**What steps should you take if you want to get tested**</u>?

Testing for COVID-19 is currently limited to people who have been exposed to SARS-CoV-2, the official name for the novel coronavirus, or who have certain symptoms, like those outlined above.

Call your doctor's office if you suspect you've contracted SARS-CoV-2. Your doctor or nurse can assess your health status and risks over the phone. They can then direct you as to how and where to go for testing, and help guide you to the right type of care.

On April 21, the Food and Drug Administration approved the use of the first COVID-19 home testing kit. Using the cotton swab provided, people will be able to collect a nasal sample and mail it to a designated laboratory for testing.

The emergency use authorization specifies that the test kit is authorized for use by people whom healthcare professionals have identified as having suspected COVID-19.

What is involved with the testing?

Polymerase chain reaction (PRC) testing remains the primary COVID-19 diagnostic testing method in the United States. This is the same type of test that was used to detect severe acute respiratory syndrome (SARS) when it first appeared in 2002.

To collect a sample for this test, a healthcare provider will likely perform one of the following:

- swab your nose or the back of your throat
- aspirate fluid from your lower respiratory tract
- take a saliva or stool sample

Researchers then extract nucleic acid from the virus sample and amplify parts of its genome through a reverse transcription PCR (RT-PCR) technique. This essentially gives them a larger sample for viral comparison. Two genes can be found within the SARS-CoV-2 genome.

Test results are:

- positive if both genes are found
- inconclusive if only one gene is found
- negative if neither gene is found

Your doctor may also order a chest CT scan to help diagnose COVID-19 or get a clearer view of how and where the virus has spread.

How long does it take to get test results?

RT-PCR samples are often tested in batches at sites away from where they were collected. This means it can take a day or longer to get test results.

The newly approved point-of-care testing allows for samples to be collected and tested at the same location, resulting in quicker turn around times.

Cepheid point-of-care devices produce test results within 45 minutes.

Is the test accurate?

In the majority of cases, RT-PCR test results are accurate. The results may not flesh out infection if tests are run too early in the disease course. The viral load may be too low to detect infection at this point.

A recent COVID-19 study found that accuracy varied, depending on when and how samples were collected.

The same study also found that chest CT scans accurately identified infection in 98 percent of cases whereas RT-PCR tests detected it correctly 71 percent of the time.

The RT-PCR may still be the most accessible test, so talk with your healthcare provider about your options if you have concerns about testing.

Part Six
Conversational English Functions

* Hesitation and Looking for the Right Words 犹豫和寻找合适的表达

Um/Uh/Er ...

Well, let me see, it's ...

It's like this, you see, ...

... , what I mean is ...

... , as a matter of fact/in fact/actually, ...

Oh yes, we-well, that's to say ...

... , how can I put it, ...

... , just let me get it right/let's see now/just a moment, oh yes, ...

... , hang on a second/I've nearly got it, ...

I'll have to think about it.

That's ... , well, what I'm trying to say is, ...

I can't think of the right words, but you know what I mean.

It's coming to me ...

I can't remember ... It's slipped my mind. You know, ...

It's on the tip of my tongue. You know what I mean.

I've forgotten what the ... is called. It's at the back of my mind.

I can't think of the exact words, but you know.

I'm not sure how I can put it.

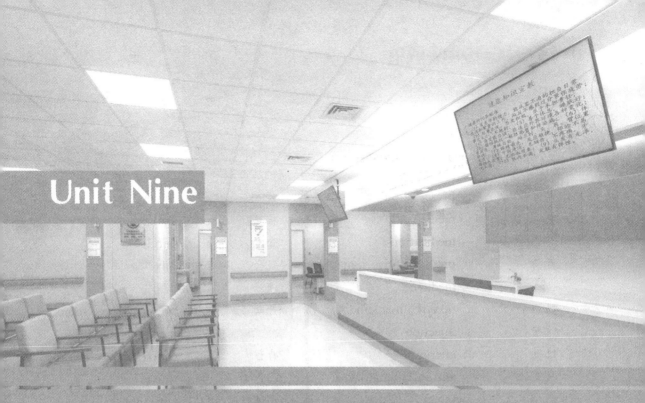

Unit Nine

Treatment Ⅰ
治疗(1)

Learning Objectives

掌握与各类药物、药效与服用方式相关的词汇及表达

掌握与药物治疗相关的句式结构

熟悉与各类辅助治疗、安慰病人相关的表达

Outline

Part One   Words and Expressions

Part Two   Model Dialogues

Part Three   Exercises

Part Four   Other Structures

Part Five   Supplementary Reading：Learn about Medications

Part Six   Conversational English Functions

      •   Interrupting

✓音、视频资源

✓参考答案

✓学术探讨

Part One

Words and Expressions

处方	prescription	吸入	inhale from
药,药物	medicine/	摇晃	shake
	medication	含漱	gargle
开药	prescribe/give some	混合	mix
	medicine	滴	drip
服药	take the medicine	开药	prescribe/give some
注射	injection		medicine
过敏	allergy	疗程	course
抗炎的	anti-inflammatory	副作用	side effect
药片	tablet	抗过敏的	anti-allergic
泡腾片	water/effervescent	药粉	powder
	tablet	药丸	pill
胶囊	capsule	药膏,软膏	ointment/cream
搽剂,涂抹油	liniment	凝胶	gel
乳液	lotion	喷雾剂	spray/nebulizer
酊剂	tincture	吸入器	inhaler
含片	lozenge	栓剂	suppository
(眼/鼻/耳)药水	(eye/nasal/ear)	糊剂	paste
	drop	抗生素	antibiotic(s)/anti-
膏剂	plaster		inflammatory(-ries)
镇静剂	sedative	抗酸药	antacid
咳嗽药水/糖浆	cough mixture/	口服药液	oral liquid medicine
	syrup	退烧药	antipyretic
肌肉松弛剂	a muscle relaxant	止吐剂	antiemetic
安眠药	sleeping pill	压,碾碎	crush
涂	apply	嚼碎,咀嚼	chew
吞	swallow	吸食	suck

按摩，揉匀	rub in/on	放置	place
塞入	insert	溶解	dissolve

Part Two

Model Dialogues

Insomnia 失眠

Patient：What about the sleeping problems?

病人：我最近的睡眠问题怎么办？

Doctor：**I'm going to prescribe you some medicine to help you get a better night's sleep.**

医生：我会给您开点药助睡眠。

Patient：Thank you, doctor.

病人：谢谢医生。

Doctor：**Here is the prescription. You can get this order at the pharmacy.**

医生：这是取药单。您可以在药房取药。

Patient：How often should I take the medicine?

病人：我多久吃一次药？

Doctor：**You can take one pill about 30 minutes before you go to bed.**

医生：睡前30分钟吃一颗。

Patient：How long should I take them?

病人：吃多久呢？

Doctor：**The prescription is for thirty days.** If you're not sleeping well after thirty days, I'd like you to come back.

医生：这是30天的量。如果30天后睡眠还是不太好，我建议您再来看看。

Patient：Is there any side effect?

病人：这药有副作用吗？

Doctor：**Common side effects may include headache, dizziness and other symptoms. Do not overdose it.**

医生：一般副作用可能包含头疼、头晕或者其他一些症状。不要过量服用。

Patient：Is there anything else I can do to help me sleep at night? Should I stay home from work?

病人：我晚上还需要做什么帮助睡眠吗？我应该留家里不上班吗？

Doctor：No, I don't think that's necessary. Just remember to stay calm.

医生：不用，没必要。尽量保持平静。

Trauma 创伤

Patient：What medicine should I take? I hope I will recover as soon as possible.

病人：我该服什么药呢？我希望能尽快痊愈。

Doctor：**I'm going to prescribe you some painkillers，antibiotics and the ointment for external use. Are you allergic to any drugs**?

医生：我给您开些止痛药、抗生素和外用药膏。您对什么药过敏吗？

Patient：Never. How should I take them?

病人：从来不过敏。这些药怎么用？

Doctor：**Please take the antibiotics two tablets each time and twice a day**, and the painkillers two pills when you need them. **The maximum dose is 4 pills a day.**

医生：抗生素每天2次，每次2片；止痛药你需要的时候服用2粒，最大剂量一天4粒。

Patient：What is the ointment used for?

病人：药膏有什么功效？

Doctor：**The ointment is also used to relieve pain. You can use it whenever you need to.**

医生：药膏可以缓解疼痛。你需要的时候可以随时涂。

Patient：Is there any side effect with the medicines?

病人：这些药有什么副作用吗？

Doctor：**You may feel discomfort with your stomach.**

医生：胃可能会有些不舒服。

Patient：How long should I take the antibiotics?

病人：抗生素需要服用多久？

Doctor：**Seven days for one course.**

医生：一个疗程是 7 天。

Patient：Where can I get them?

病人：在哪里拿药？

Doctor：You can go to the pharmacy. It's not far away from here.

医生：去药房取药，离这里不远。

Patient：What else should I do for my recovery?

病人：我还需要怎么做才能早点康复？

Doctor：**No seafood. Keep a light diet.**

医生：不要吃海鲜。饮食尽量清淡。

Patient：Is it serious?

病人：我的伤算严重吗？

Doctor：**Don't worry, and everything will be OK soon.**

医生：别担心，很快就会好的。

Useful Structures

1. I'm going to prescribe/give you some medicine to（help you get a better night's sleep）.

    我会给您开点药（助睡眠）。

2. I'm going to prescribe/give you some painkillers, antibiotics and the ointment for external use.

    我给您开些止痛药、抗生素和外用药膏。

3. Here is the prescription. You can get this order at the pharmacy.

    这是取药单。您可以在药房取药。

4. You can take one pill about 30 minutes before you go to bed.

    睡前 30 分钟吃一颗。

5. The prescription is for（thirty）days.

    这是（30）天的量。

6. （Seven）days for one course.

    一个疗程（7）天。

7. Common side effects may include headache, dizziness and other symptoms.

Do not overdose it.

副作用可能包含头疼、头晕或者其他一些症状。不要过量服用。

8. Are you allergic to any drugs?

您对什么药过敏吗?

9. Please take the antibiotics two tablets each time and twice a day.

抗生素每天2次,每次2颗。

10. The maximum dose is (4 pills) a day.

最大剂量是每天(4粒)。

11. The ointment is used to relieve the pain.

药膏可以缓解疼痛。

12. You can use it whenever you need to.

您需要的时候随时可以使用。

13. You may feel discomfort with(your stomach).

(胃)可能会有些不舒服。

14. No seafood. Keep a light diet.

不要吃海鲜。饮食尽量清淡。

15. Don't worry, and everything will be OK soon.

别担心,很快就会好的。

Part Three

Exercises

- Put the following sentences or short conversations into English.

1. 吞下药片_____

2. 碾碎药丸成粉状_____

3. 将药粉与水混合_____

4. 将药膏涂抹在皮肤上_____

5. 使用前摇匀_____

6. 将药膏按摩揉匀_____

7. 将混合液滴入糖管_____

8. 将混合液每天含漱三次_____

9. 从吸入剂中吸入_____

10. 患病期间避免吃油腻食品_____

11. 不要吃豆类食品_____

12. 病人:我该去哪里拿药?

_____

医生:去药房取药。

_____

病人:这药要服用多久?

_____

医生:一个疗程是 7 天。每天最多吃 6 片。

_____

13. 病人:请问我需要服用什么药呢?

_____

医生:我给你开些退烧药降体温(bring down)。

_____

病人:会有什么副作用吗?

_____

医生:一般不会。只有胃可能会有些不舒服。

_____

14. 医生:我给你开些胃药。

_____

病人:谢谢。这个胃药有什么功效?

_____

医生:这是用来中和胃酸的(neutralize acid)。

_____

病人:我怎么服用呢?

_____

医生:饭前吃,每次一颗,每天三次。

_____

病人:我要吃多久?

医生：这是四星期的量。如果没有好转再来复诊。

- Complete the following dialogue according to the instructions.

Patient：What medicine do I get?

Doctor：_____ . (cough mixture)

Patient：Is there any side effect?

Doctor：Generally speaking, there would be no side effect. Maybe _____

_____ . (stomach)

Patient：How should I take it?

Doctor：_____ . (shake)

Patient：How often should I take it?

Doctor：_____ . (amount and times)

Patient：Where can I get the mixture?

Doctor：_____ . (1st floor)

Patient：What else should I do for my recovery?

Doctor：_____ . (rest and sleep)

Patient：Is it serious?

Doctor：_____ . (making comforts)

Part Four

Other Structures

1. Be sure to take it according to the instructions. /Be sure to follow the instructions.

    请按说明书指示服药。

2. This is your prescription.

    这是您的处方。

3. I'm going to give/prescribe you a course of (tablets, antibiotics).

    我会给您开一疗程的(药片、抗生素)。

4. I'll prescribe something else that wouldn't cause you any allergic reactions.

我会另给您开些您不会过敏的药。

5. I'll prescribe you some medicine to alleviate your symptoms.

我会给您开点药减轻您的症状。

6. This medicine is used for candida infection.

这药用于念珠菌感染。

7. This medicine is used to relieve pain/eliminate the infection/neutralize acid in the stomach/bring the temperature down/bring the blood pressure down/ treat bronchial asthma/dilate blood vessels and improve circulation.

这个药用于减轻疼痛/消除感染/中和胃酸/降温/降压/治疗哮喘/扩张血管和改善血液循环。

8. The side effects are greater than the curative ones.

副作用大于疗效。

9. It's rather difficult to treat.

这种病很难治疗。

10. We can treat it by (injection/operation).

我们可以(注射/手术)治疗。

11. You need an (epinephrine) injection.

您需要注射(肾上腺素)。

12. Aspirin sometimes affects the stomach. I think you may switch into/could take/have an alternative choice, by taking Paracetamol instead.

阿司匹林对胃有副作用。我觉得您可以换成对乙酰氨基酚。

13. I'll adjust the dosage of your pill.

我会调整您药的用量。

14. I'll give you a complete dosage of one month.

我会给您开一个月的剂量。

15. You'll have to take one capsule three times a day, preferably immediately after meals.

这个胶囊每天服用 3 次,每次 1 颗,最好饭后立刻服用。

16. Take it twice a day, and 200 milliliters/2 teaspoons each time.

每日 2 次,每次 200 毫升/2 茶匙。

17. Take it once every 4 hours or more.

间隔 4 小时或以上服用。

18. You need to take this medicine orally/sublingually/anally/as a patch/as an inhalant.

您需要口服/舌下含服/肛敷/外敷/口喷。

19. Drip three drops into the affected.

将药滴三滴在患处。

20. Please take this sub-lingual tablets when you are in pain. Put it under your tongue and wait for it to dissolve.

当你觉得疼的时候,请服用这些含片,含在舌下让它自动融化。

21. Don't be nervous. You'll recover soon.

别紧张。很快就会康复了。

22. Don't do too much work/stress yourself out and avoid catching a cold.

不能劳累,避免受凉。

23. Eat lightly.

饮食要清淡。

24. Take fluids. Lactose/sugar free.

喝流质。不含乳糖/糖。

25. Drink more water to protect yourself from sunstroke.

多喝水防止中暑。

26. Eat more food rich in Vitamin C such as vegetables and fruits. Keep a diet of low fat and low sugar.

多吃富含维生素 C 的食物,比如蔬菜、水果。饮食要低脂低糖。

27. Wash your hands more frequently, avoid touching your eyes with your hands and do not share your towel with others.

勤洗手,避免用手摸眼以及与他人共用毛巾。

Part Five

Supplementary Reading：Learn about Medications

Medications are drugs manufactured to help people deal with a range of health issues. Some medications are psychoactive (mind altering) while others are not.

Some medications—for colds, flus, headaches and stomachaches—are sold over the counter and therefore do not require a prescription. Medications that are prescribed include the following:

- antibiotics (for bacterial infections)
- antidepressants (for depression)
- cardiovascular drugs (for heart disease)
- opiates (for pain)
- stimulants (for attention deficit hyperactivity disorder)
- tranquilizers and sleeping pills (for stress, anxiety and sleeping problems)

Medications usually come as pills or tablets and are swallowed or administered as suppositories. Some medications come in liquid form and can be injected. Other medications come in slips that fit under the tongue and dissolve in the mouth. Medications can be short-, medium-, or long-acting, referring to the length of time the drug affects the body.

Why do we use medications?

We use medications to relieve symptoms of medical conditions, to combat both short-term and chronic illness, and to manage our daily lives. While medications may be beneficial, they can also be harmful.

Using a medication to treat pain can be helpful. But over time, we may become tolerant to the drug and need an increasing amount to feel the positive effects. Some medications, such as tranquilizers, may help to relieve stress, but relying on a substance as a tool to ease tension can affect our health and relationships. And while using a medication as instructed or prescribed can help us manage our health, taking more than the recommended dosage can harm our health.

What happens when we use medications?

Different medications affect the brain and body in different ways. For example, stimulant medications speed up activity in the central nervous system while depressant medications, such as tranquilizers, slow down activity in the brain. Pain medications block pain receptors in the brain, thereby decreasing the amount of pain felt. And antibiotics treat bacterial infections by killing the bacteria or preventing it from multiplying.

The way a particular form of medication affects us depends on more than just the type, dosage and method of administration. Other factors include our:

- past experiences with the drug,
- present mood and circumstances,
- weight and age, and
- use (or non-use) of other drugs at the same time.

Health effects

When we think of medications, we normally think of them as tools for getting better. We may not be aware there can be harms as well as benefits. For instance, our doctor may prescribe a sleeping pill to help us get our sleeping pattern back on track. But after a few weeks of regular use, we may develop tolerance to the sleep-inducing effects and, if we continue to take higher doses, may find it hard to stop using the drug. And many medications can cause side effects. For instance, tranquilizers affect psychomotor coordination and, as a result, driving ability is impaired.

Medications can also have an impact on our social, school and work lives. For instance, if we combine alcohol with some medications such as tranquilizers, the effects of both drugs are increased. This can put us at risk of making bad decisions such as having unprotected driving before the effects have worn off. Some medications affect our ability to remember and learn things. This could impair our ability to do well in school or perform at work.

Some people use medications over the long term because they find the drugs helpful for managing ongoing health problems. For instance, a person may require cardiovascular drugs to control blood pressure or opiates to address chronic pain. But it is important to remember that making good decisions about using medications involves regular consultations with a healthcare professional and weighing the benefits and risks of continuing use.

Remember, not all bugs need drugs. Not all problems need drugs either. Other healthy ways to feel better include exercise, good diet and enough sleep.

When is using medication a problem?

Using a medication is a problem when it negatively affects our life or the lives of others. For instance, it can be risky to use some medications for too long or in certain contexts, such as when drinking alcohol or when pregnant. What's important is to be aware of the potential benefits and harms related to using the medication in various contexts and over time.

A number of us, particularly those who are older, may be prescribed several medications. But when we mix some medications, we may be putting ourselves at risk of harm. Using an opiate and a sleeping pill, for example, can magnify the drowsiness effects of both drugs, potentially leading to harmful consequences such as becoming overly sedated.

Sometimes medications are used in ways not intended or prescribed. For instance, taking more than the recommended dosage, using someone else's prescription medication, and using medications for non-medical purposes are all risky. When we use medications in these ways, we are potentially putting ourselves at risk for adverse consequences.

When using medications, carefully read the labels and any accompanying information. Discuss any concerns with your healthcare professional, and seek advice if you are considering no longer using a medication. People who stop using some medications after regular use can experience feelings of withdrawal, including irritability, loss of appetite and difficulty sleeping. These are usually temporary, but consult your healthcare provider if problems persist.

Mixing substances

People sometimes use more than one medication at a time or mix medications with other substances without realizing there is potential for harmful consequences. For example, someone may drink alcohol with an opiate painkiller without understanding that using these depressant drugs together can be harmful. Some interactions may be minor, but others can be dangerous and possibly life threatening. The following are possible effects when drugs are combined.

They may act independently of one another. For example, antibiotics do not seem to interfere with tranquilizers such as benzodiazepines (e. g., Valium and

Ativan).

They may increase each other's effects. For example, mixing opiates and tranquilizers (both slow the central nervous system) could result in reducing blood pressure and breathing rates to dangerous levels.

They may decrease each other's intended effects. For instance, tobacco smoke interacts with some medications and people who smoke may require higher doses.

How to make healthier choices about medications

Whenever we decide to use medications, it is helpful to know what steps we can take to ensure that our use results in the most benefit with the least harm. The following are some useful guidelines to follow.

Not too much. Always follow the dose instructions and remember that using more than one medication at a time may be risky.

Tip: Always ask your healthcare professional if there are other drugs (including alcohol) to avoid while using a particular medication.

Not too often. Using a drug more frequently than prescribed or for longer than recommended may be dangerous.

Tip: Check with your healthcare professional if you are not feeling the positive effects of a medication.

Only in safe contexts. Making informed decisions about situations where a medication may reduce your ability to function safely and responsibly helps to minimize harms.

Tip: Always read the label and other information provided with the medication. Check for warnings concerning the effects on physical and mental functioning (e. g., driving ability).

Are all medications legal?

All over-the-counter medications sold in reputable stores are legal. Prescription medications are legal when prescribed by an authorized healthcare professional. Using someone else's prescription or selling prescribed medication to other people is illegal.

Part Six

Conversational English Functions

• Interrupting 打断

1. Interrupting Politely

Can I say something here?

I'd like to say/add something, if I may.

If I could just come in here ...

Sorry to interrupt, but ...

Can I add something?

Can I interrupt you for a moment?

I'd just like to say that ...

Excuse me for interrupting, but ...

That reminds me ...

Can I ask a question?

May I ask something?

Sorry, but ...

2. Preventing Interruptions or Bringing the Discussion Back to the Original Topic

There are two/three points I'd like to make ...

Although ...

And another thing ...

To return to the topic ...

Anyway ...

To get back to what I was saying ...

Where was I?

Would you mind waiting till I finish?

Just a minute, please.

Can you wait for a while, please?

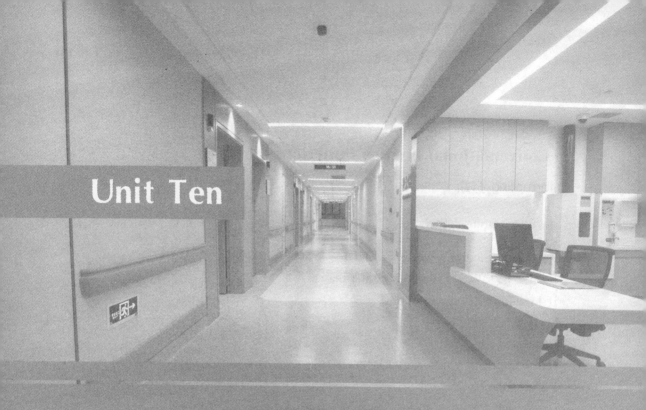

Unit Ten

Treatment Ⅱ
治疗(2)

Learning Objectives

熟悉各类外伤的英文名称

熟悉与各类外伤治疗方法相关的词汇及表达

掌握与外伤治疗方法及目的相关的句型结构

掌握急救相关用语

Outline

Part One   Words and Expressions

Part Two   Model Dialogues

Part Three Exercises

Part Four   Other Structures

Part Five   Supplementary Reading：Cardiopulmonary

Resuscitation（CPR）：First Aid

Part Six   Conversational English Functions

• Intention

✓音、视频资源

✓参考答案

✓学术探讨

Part One

Words and Expressions

折断(骨折)	fracture/fractured
拉伤	sprain/sprained
跛(的)	cripple/crippled
弯曲(的)	bend/bent
韧带	ligament
支撑绷	support bandage
石膏(固定敷料)	plaster cast
夹板	splint
腿部固定器；腿部支架	leg brace
护腹器	abdominal protector
止血带	tourniquet
止血	stop bleeding
固定	set/fix (your bone/limb)
骨折固定术	fracture fixation
作业治疗	occupational therapy/OT
冰敷	compress with ice/ice it
扭伤	twist/twisted
脱臼	dislocation/dislocated
突出,凸起(的)	protrusion/protruding
畸形,变形	deformity
绷带	bandage
三角绷带	triangle bandage
悬臂板	back slab
颈托	neck support
护腹带	support abdominal bandage
手部固定器	hand fixator
包扎(伤口)	bandage up (the wound)
缝针	stitch up (the wound)
抬高	keep ... elevated
物理治疗	physiotherapy/PT
止血法	hemostasis
纱布	gauze

Part Two

Model Dialogues

Fracture 骨折

Doctor：I'm afraid your elbow might be broken. I think you need to have an X-ray of your elbow.

医生：可能您的肘部骨折了。肘部需要照 X 光。

Patient：OK. Sure.

病人：好的。

After the test 化验之后

Patient：Here is my X-ray image.

病人：这是我的 X 光片。

Doctor：Let me have a look. Well，**the X-ray shows that your elbow is fractured. You need to apply a U-shaped plaster cast over your elbow and shoulder to fix the fracture.**

医生：我看看。X 光片显示您的肘部骨折。您的肘部、肩部需要用 U 型石膏固定骨折部位。

Patient：Is it serious?

病人：很严重吗?

Doctor：Don't worry. Nothing serious.

医生：不严重。别担心。

Patient：How long will I have to wear it?

病人：我需要固定多久?

Doctor：**I'm afraid you must wear it for about six weeks.**

医生：恐怕需要 6 星期左右。

Patient：What else should I do?

病人：还有什么其他需要注意的地方吗?

Doctor：Rest in bed and try to keep your elbow elevated above your heart as much as possible.

医生：尽量卧床，将肘部抬起到心脏部位，越高越好。

Patient：Why?

病人：为什么要这样？

Doctor：**It helps the blood return to your heart and helps to reduce the swelling. Do not hesitate to check in whenever there is a problem**，such as aggravated pain or numbness of the arm，hand or fingers. I'll check if the fixation is in position or not.

医生：这样可以帮助血液流向心脏以降低肿胀的可能。一有问题就来找我，比如疼痛加强，手臂、手或手指发麻。我会检查看石膏有没有固定好。

Patient：Do I need to take the medicine?

病人：我需要服药吗？

Doctor：Yes. I'll prescribe you some painkillers to relieve the pain.

医生：我会给您开些止痛药缓解疼痛。

Patient：Doctor, do I have osteoporosis(骨质疏松)?

病人：医生，我有骨质疏松吗？

Doctor：**You will need more tests to make the diagnosis.**

医生：您需要更多的检查才能确诊是否有骨质疏松。

Six weeks later 6 周后

Doctor：**I'm pleased to say that your fracture has healed in a very good position and now I need to take the cast off.**

医生：非常高兴告诉您，您的骨折已经治愈了，现在我要把石膏解下。

Patient：So wonderful! Thank you very much，doctor.

病人：太棒了。非常感谢您，医生。

Doctor：It's done. You may go now.

医生：好了。您现在可以走了。

Patient：OK! Bye!

病人：好的！再见！

Doctor：Bye!

医生：再见！

Useful Structures

1. The X-ray shows that your elbow is fractured.

   X 光显示您肘部骨折。

2. You need to apply a U-shaped plaster cast over your elbow and shoulder to fix the fracture.

   您的肘部、肩部需要用 U 型石膏固定骨折部位。

3. I'm afraid you must wear it for about six weeks.

   恐怕需要 6 星期左右。

4. It helps the blood return to your heart and helps to reduce the swelling.

   这样可以帮助血液流向心脏以降低肿胀的可能。

5. Do not hesitate to check in whenever there is a problem.

   一有问题就来找我。

6. You will need more tests to make the diagnosis.

   您需要更多的检查才能确诊是否有骨质疏松。

7. I'm pleased to say that your fracture has healed in a very good position and now I need to take the cast off.

   非常高兴告诉您,您的骨折已经治愈了,现在我要把石膏解下。

Emergency 急救

Receptionist：Paramedic 127. **What's the address of your emergency**?

接线员：救援中心 127 号机线员。请问您的求救地址是哪里?

Man：Help! Help! **I need an ambulance.**

男士：求救求救! 我需要一辆救护车。

Receptionist：OK，Sir! What's the address?

接线员：好的,先生! 请问您的地址是什么?

Man：I'm not sure. I think it's King Street. I need an ambulance.

男士：我不太确定。应该是国王大街吧。我需要一辆救护车。

Receptionist：Sir, **we'll get to help right away**.

接线员：先生,我们马上就会去进行救援。

Man：Please hurry! Hurry! **Can you send an ambulance**?

男士:赶快赶快！能派遣救护车吗？

Receptionist：OK，Sir! **What's the nature of the emergency**?

接线员:好的,先生！是什么急症？

Man：My son is lying here. He's not conscious. He is not moving.

男士:我儿子躺在这里。他没意识了。他动不了。

Receptionist：OK! He is not moving. He's unconscious.

接线员:好的！他动不了。他失去意识了。

Man：Right.

男士:好的。

Receptionist：OK，Sir! **An ambulance is on the way.** It will be a few minutes. Did you see what happened to your son?

接线员:好的,先生！救护车正赶往救援。大概几分钟时间。请问您看见您儿子发生了什么吗？

Man：He was riding his bike，and it crashed to a tree.

男士:他骑自行车撞到了大树上。

Receptionist：OK，Sir! **I've dispatched all the information to the paramedics.**

接线员:好的,先生。我们已经把所有信息传递给救护人员了。

Man：Thank you!

男士:谢谢！

A moment later 一会以后

Man：Thank you for your help. Is it serious?

男士:谢谢您的帮助！他的伤严重吗？

Paramedics：**We need to send him to the hospital right away for further examination. Do you agree**?

救护人员:我们需要立刻把他送到医院作进一步检查。您同意吗？

Man：Sure! Thank you very much.

男士:当然可以！非常感谢！

After the patient is awake 病人醒来后

Doctor：Alright，Sir. Don't panic. You've just had a terrible accident and you're in the emergency room at Moonlight Hospital.

医生：好的，先生。不要慌张。您出了交通意外现在在月光医院的急诊室。

Patient：What? Where am I? I don't remember anything. Who are you?

病人：什么？我在哪儿？我什么也记不清了。您是谁？

Doctor：I'm Doctor Smith.

医生：我是史密斯医生。

Patient：What happened? Why am I here?

病人：发生了什么？我怎么在这儿？

Doctor：Well，you crashed your bike into a tree and lost your consciousness. You've broken your arm. But don't worry. We'll take good care of you.

医生：好吧，您骑车撞在大树上了，失去了意识，并且胳膊也摔断了。不过，不要紧。我们会好好照顾您的。

Patient：What are you going to do?

病人：那您现在要怎么处理？

Doctor：Now I need you to relax. We are going to give you some painkillers to help you feel better.

医生：现在需要您休息一下。我们将给您服用一些止痛药让您舒适一些。

Patient：Pain? What pain? I don't feel anything in my arm.

病人：痛？什么痛？我胳膊没感觉到什么疼痛。

Doctor：OK. **That's not good. We have to start operating immediately.** Please don't move and keep quiet.

医生：这个情况不太好。我们必须立刻给您手术。请不要动，保持安静。

Patient：OK, doctor. **I'll do my best.**

病人：好的，医生。我会尽力的。

Two hours later 两小时后

Doctor：Hello? Hello! Are you awake? Can you see me?

医生：您好！您苏醒了吗？可以看见我吗？

Patient：Yes. I can see you.

病人：可以。我看得见你。

Doctor：Do you feel any pain in your arm?

医生：您的胳膊感觉到痛了吗?

Patient：Ouch! That hurts.

病人：啊! 很疼。

Doctor：Great! **The operation was a success**! We had to reattach the nerves that were injured during your accident. You'll have to rest for two months. **And in order to heal I recommend that you do not play any sports or use your cell phone for the next two months.** You may go now. Goodbye!

医生：太棒了。手术很成功! 我们不得不将事故中您受伤的神经重新接上。您必须再休息2个月时间。为了您能尽快恢复,在此期间,我建议您不要进行任何体育运动或者用手机。您现在就可以出院了。再见!

Patient：Thank you，doctor. Goodbye!

病人：谢谢医生。再见!

Useful Structures

1. What's the address of your emergency?

   请问您的求救地址是哪里?

2. We'll get to help right away.

   我们马上就会去进行救援。

3. Can you send an ambulance?

   能派遣救护车吗?

4. What's the nature of the emergency?

   是什么样的急症?

5. An ambulance is on the way.

   救护车正赶往救援。

6. I've dispatched all the information to the paramedics.

   我们已经把所有信息传递给救护人员。

7. We need to send him to the hospital right away for further examination. Do you agree?

   我们需要立刻把他送到医院做进一步检查。您同意吗?

8. That's not good. We have to start operating immediately.
    这个情况不太好。我们必须立刻给您做手术。

9. I'll do my best.
    我会尽力的。

10. The operation was a success!
    手术很成功!

11. And in order to heal I recommend that you do not play any sports or use your cell phone for the next two months.
    为了您能尽快恢复,在接下来两个月内,我建议您不要进行任何体育运动或者用手机。

Part Three
Exercises

- Put the following sentences or short conversations into English.

1. 您的腿(可能)拉伤了。

    _____

2. X 光片显示您的胳膊脱臼了。

    _____

3. 您需要绑石膏。

    _____

4. 您的膝盖需要用夹板固定。

    _____

5. 您的腿需要冰敷。

    _____

6. 这三天您必须尽量抬高脚。

    _____

7. 这是止血带,可以防止进一步出血。

    _____

8. 这是颈托,以防止您的颈椎进一步损伤。

_____

9. 非常高兴告诉您,您的扭伤已经好了。

_____

10. 您的伤口很大,我会给您缝针。

_____

11. 医生：X 光片显示您的腿部没有骨折。

_____

病人:太好了! 那接下来我该怎么小?

_____

医生:您需要多休息。回去 48 小时内用冰敷。如果一直不见好转或情况恶化,再来医院复查。

_____

12. 医生:我们要对您进行止血,包扎,固定。

_____

病人:好的,伤口很严重吗?

_____

医生:放轻松,都会好的。现在我们需要把您送到指定医院做进一步检查,好吗?

_____

- **Complete the following dialogue according to the instructions.**

Now that you've learned a complete process of inquiry in English, please complete the following dialogues according to the Chinese given below or the answers from the patient.

1. Injury 受伤

Doctor: _____?

Patient: I think I've twisted my ankle. /My ankle is twisted.

Doctor: _____. (我需要检查一下您的脚。)

Patient: OK.

Doctor: _____?

Patient：It hurts here.

Doctor：＿＿＿＿＿＿＿＿＿＿＿＿＿＿＿＿＿＿＿＿＿＿＿＿＿？

Patient：I slipped down some stairs.

Doctor：＿＿＿＿＿＿＿＿＿＿＿＿＿＿＿＿＿＿＿＿＿？（疼得厉害吗？）

Patient：Very severe.

Doctor：Can you move now?

Patient：No，not really. It hurts if I do.

Doctor：＿＿＿＿＿＿＿＿＿＿＿＿＿＿＿＿＿＿＿？（你的脚肿了吗？）

Patient：Yes, I think so. My foot is swollen but my toes are not.

Doctor：＿＿＿＿＿＿＿＿＿＿＿＿＿＿＿＿？（你的脚趾有知觉吗？）

Patient：Yes.

Doctor：＿＿＿＿＿＿＿＿＿＿＿＿＿＿＿＿＿＿＿＿＿＿＿＿＿＿＿

＿＿＿＿＿＿＿＿＿＿＿＿＿？（你有刺痛的感觉吗？还是觉得麻？）

Patient：No. To be honest, it hurts too much for me to notice anything else.

Doctor：＿＿＿＿＿＿＿＿＿＿＿＿＿＿＿＿＿＿.（你需要拍下 X 光。）

Patient：How could I find it?

Doctor：＿＿＿＿＿＿＿＿＿＿＿＿＿＿＿＿＿＿＿＿＿＿＿＿＿＿＿

＿＿＿＿＿＿＿.（在 2 楼。出门左拐一直走,在你右手边就可以看到楼梯口。）

Patient：OK. Thank you very much.

Doctor：＿＿＿＿＿＿＿＿＿＿＿＿＿＿＿＿.（拿到 X 光片以后带过来找我。）

Patient：Do I have to wait for it?

Doctor：Yes.

Doctor：I have seen your X-ray. ＿＿＿＿＿＿＿＿＿＿＿＿＿＿＿＿

＿＿＿＿＿＿＿＿＿＿＿＿＿＿＿＿.（片子显示没有骨折。）

Patient：Thank goodness.

Doctor：＿＿＿＿＿＿＿＿＿＿＿＿＿＿＿＿＿＿＿＿＿.［你

需要绑下（支撑）绷带。3 天内或者你症状好转前,尽量让你的脚抬着。］

Patient：OK.

Doctor：＿＿＿＿＿＿＿＿＿＿＿＿＿＿＿＿＿＿＿＿＿＿＿＿＿＿＿

＿＿＿＿＿＿＿＿＿＿＿.（如果一个星期后脚踝还没有好转再来找我。）

2. Diarrhea 腹泻

Doctor：_____？（你的粪便是什么样子的？）

Patient：Light brown and watery stool.

Doctor：_____？（有气味吗？）

Patient：They usually smell.

Doctor：_____？（腹泻时有痛感吗？）

Patient：Yes，just before I want to go to the toilet.

Doctor：_____？（是什么样的痛呢？）

Patient：It's a kind of griping pain.

Doctor：_____？（哪儿痛呢？）

Patient：I have a pain in my lower stomach. Here.

Doctor：_____.

（我需要给你做下检查。我要按下你的肚子，你感到疼的时候就告诉我。）

Patient：Right here.

Doctor：_____？（有多强烈？）

Patient：I think it's mild.

Doctor：_____？（呕吐吗？）

Patient：No.

Doctor：Do you think it was something you ate?

Patient：I did wonder if it was something I ate，but it's been 4 days now，normally if it was something I ate，it would have stopped by now.

Doctor：_____？（服用过药物吗？）

Patient：No，I haven't taken any medicine recently.

Doctor：_____？（你现在能吃得进东西吗？）

Patient：No，not really. I try to eat something but it goes straight through me.

Doctor：_____？（能喝流质吗？）

Patient：Yes，I am taking fluids.

Doctor：_____？（你感到虚弱头晕吗？）

Patient：No，not really.

Doctor：_____？（你是否感到发烧或者头痛？）

Patient：No.

Doctor：_____?

Patient：I do feel a bit dehydrated，but I have been trying to take fluids.

Doctor：_____

_____.（我需要一些你的粪便样本，这是样本瓶。你还需要做一下血液检查，拍 X 光以及超声波扫描。）

Patient：Where do I have to go?

Doctor：_____

_____.（护士会带你过去，你拿到结果后再来找我。）

Patient：Thanks.

Doctor：_____.（你的化验报告表明你食物中毒导致肠部感染，你的 X 光和扫描结果都很正常。）

Patient：Oh，so I do have food poisoning. Is it serious?

Doctor：_____.（放轻松，不严重。）

Patient：Do I need any medication?

Doctor：_____.（对。我会给你开些抗生素口服。这是处方。）

Patient：Where can I get them?

Doctor：_____.（去药房拿药，药房在 1 楼。）

Patient：Oh，OK. How and how long do I take it?

Doctor：_____.

（按说明书上指示服用。3 天一个疗程。）

Patient：What else should I do for my recovery at home?

Doctor：_____.（多喝流质，好转前饮食尽量清淡。多休息。）

Patient：Thank you.

Doctor：_____.（如果没有好转再来找我。）

Part Four

Other Structures

1. Our ambulance will send you to the Emergency Department of the designated hospital.

我们的救护车会将您送到指定医院的急诊科。

2. We have limited facilities so you have to go to the hospital for further examination. Do you agree? If you refuse to go, your problem may get worse.

我们这里治疗手段有限,所以您需要去医院做进一步检查。您同意吗? 如果您不去的话,病情可能会加重。

3. If you don't agree to go to the hospital，you need to sign for this on your clinical record.

如果你拒绝去医院,需要在病历上写明情况并签字。

4. Your arm needs to get ... stitches.

您的手臂需要缝合……针。

5. Your arm needs to be in/have a sling; you must keep it on for ... days.

您的手臂需要悬臂板;您必须戴……天。

6. We need your cooperation.

我们需要您的配合。

7. You need an emergency treatment.

您需要紧急处理。

8. The medical guiding nurse will send a flatcar/stretcher here immediately.

导医会马上送平车/担架过来。

9. Here is the flatcar/stretcher and you can lie on it now. We will send you to the emergency department at once.

平车/担架到了,您可以躺在上面。我们立刻将您送到急诊室。

10. We must place you on a stretcher with a restraint strap, which may make you a little uncomfortable. Do you understand what I am trying to say? Are the straps too tight?

我们要用约束带将您固定在担架上,这可能有点不舒服。您明白了吗? 约束带紧吗?

11. The road maybe a little bumpy. If you feel uncomfortable on the way, please let me know.

路上可能会有些颠簸。如果您觉得不舒服,请告诉我。

12. We've arrived now. Please don't move while we are taking you out of the vehicle.

我们已经到了。我们将您抬下车,请不要动。

13. I have described your condition to the doctors who will receive you.

我已经向接诊医生交代了您的病情。

14. You should pay cash for the out-call ambulance. It is the regulation here in China. This is your receipt. Please keep it and submit it to the insurance company to get your money back.

请您结账。在中国,救护车出诊需要通过现金结账。这是您的收据。请妥善保管之后到保险公司报销。

15. Now，we must watch over you and give you oxygen.

现在我们将监护您并给您吸氧。

16. We will give you a priority to the treatment.

我们会给您安排优先就诊。

17. We'll put you under observation. It doesn't hurt to monitor you for a few hours just to make sure you're fine.

我们需要对您进行观察。这对人身体没有伤害。只是观察几小时以确保您没事。

Part Five

Supplementary Reading：Cardiopulmonary Resuscitation (CPR)：First Aid

The American Heart Association uses the letters CAB：compression, airway, breathing—to help people to remember the order to perform the steps of CPR.

Compressions：Restore blood circulation

1. Put the person on his or her back on a firm surface.

2. Kneel next to the person's neck and shoulders.

3. Place the heel of one hand over the center of the person's chest between the person's nipples. Place your other hand on top of the first hand. Keep your elbows straight and position your shoulders directly above your hands.

4. Use your upper body weight(not just your arms) as you push straight down on/compress the chest at least 2 inches(approximately 5 centimeters) but no greater than 2.4 inches(approximately 6 centimeters). Push hard at a rate of 100 to 120

compressions a minute.

5. If you haven't been trained in CPR, continue chest compressions until there are signs of movement or until emergency medical personnel take over. If you have been trained in CPR, go on opening the airway and rescue breathing.

Airway: Open the airway

If you're trained in CPR and you've performed 30 chest compressions, open the person's airway using the head-tilt, chin-lift maneuver. Put your palm on the person's forehead and gently tilt the head back. Then with the other hand, gently lift the chin forward to open the airway.

Breathing: Breathe for the person

Rescue breathing can be mouth-to-mouth breathing or mouth-to-nose breathing if the mouth is seriously injured or can't be opened.

1. With the airway open(using the head-tilt, chin-lift maneuver), pinch the nostrils shut for mouth-to-mouth breathing and cover the person's mouth with yours, making a seal.

2. Prepare to give two rescue breaths. Give the first rescue breath—lasting one second—and watch to see if the chest rises. If it does rise, give the second breath if the chest doesn't rise, repeat the head-tilt, chin-lift maneuver and then give the second breath. Thirty chest compressions followed by two rescue breaths is considered one cycle. Be careful not to provide too many breaths or to breathe with too much force.

3. Resume chest compressions to restore circulation.

4. As soon as an automated external defibrillator(AED) is available, apply it and follow the prompts. Administer one shock, then resume CPR—starting with chest compressions—for two more minutes before administering a second shock. If you're not trained to use an AED, other emergency medical operator may be able to guide you in its use. If an AED isn't available, go to step 5 below.

5. Continue CPR until there are signs of movement or emergency medical personnel take over.

Part Six

Conversational English Functions

- ## Intention 意图

1. Asking about Somebody's Intention

Are you going to ... ?

Are you thinking of ... ?

Do you reckon you'll ... ?

You'll ... , won't you?

Do you have any intention of doing ... ?

Do you intend to ... ?

What do you intend to do?

Have you decided to ... ?

What do you mean to do?

Do you plan to ... ?

Do you mean to ... ?

What do you reckon about ... ?

How do you feel about ... ?

2. Stating Your Intention

I feel inclined to ...

I mean to ...

I thought about doing ...

I'm planning to ...

I've decided to ...

I expect I'll ...

I'm figuring on ...

I'm hoping to ...

I have every intention of ...

My intention is to ...

3. Stating You Do not Intend to Do Something

I don't plan to ...

I don't feel inclined to ...

I'm not planning to ...

I've decided not to ...

It never entered my head to ...

I don't intend to ...

I'm not thinking of ...

I don't think I'll ...

It is not my intention to ...

Nothing could induce me to ...

附录 A　常见疾病名称

1. 上呼吸道感染 infection of the upper respiratory tract
2. 急性气管/支气管炎 acute trachea/bronchitis
3. 肺炎 pneumonia
4. 支气管哮喘 bronchus asthma
5. 胸腔积液 product liquid of thoracic cavity；hydrothorax
6. 急性呼吸衰竭 acute respiration failure
7. 消化不良 indigestion/dyspepsia
8. 急性胃肠炎 acute gastroenteritis
9. 胃炎/肠炎 gastritis/enteritis
10. 胃、十二指肠溃疡 stomach/duodenum ulcer
11. 上(下)消化道出血 upper(lower) gastrointestinal hemorrhage(or bleeding)
12. 肝炎 hepatitis
13. 高血压 hypertension
14. 冠心病、心绞痛、心肌梗死 coronary heart disease，angina，myocardial infarction
15. 心律失常 arrhythmia
16. 感染性心内膜炎 infective endocarditis
17. 心肌炎 myocarditis
18. 心力衰竭 heart failure
19. 心源性猝死 cardiogenic sudden death
20. 尿路感染 urinary tract infection
21. 慢性肾炎 chronic nephritis
22. 尿路结石 urinary stones/calculus(单数)/calculi(复数)
23. 急、慢性肾功能不全 acute/chronic kidney failure
24. 糖尿病 diabetes
25. 低血糖反应 hypoglycemic reaction
26. 痛风 gout

27. 酒精中毒 alcoholism/alcohol intoxication

28. 药物中毒 drug poisoning

29. 晕车/船 car sickness/ship sickness

30. 中暑 heatstroke

31. 淹溺 drowning

32. 电击 electrical stroke

33. 血管神经性头痛 vascular neurotic headache/angioneurotic headache

34. 三叉神经痛 trigeminal neuralgia

35. 偏头痛 migraine

36. 紧张性头痛 tension headache

37. 脑缺血 cerebral ischemic

38. 脑栓塞 brain embolism

39. 脑出血 cerebral hemorrhage

40. 高血压脑病 hypertensive encephalopathy

41. 脑膜炎、脑炎 meningitis，encephalitis

42. 癫痫 epilepsy

43. 感染 infection

44. 创伤 trauma

45. 烧伤 burn

46. 肋骨骨折 rib fracture

47. 气胸 pneumothorax

48. 血胸 hemothorax

49. 腹外疝 external hernia

50. 急性腹膜炎 acute peritonitis

51. 肠梗阻 intestinal obstruction/ileus

52. 急性阑尾炎 acute appendicitis

53. 胆结石 cholelithiasis/gall-stone

54. 急性胆管炎 acute cholangitis

55. 急性胆囊炎 acute cholecystitis

56. 急性胰腺炎 acute pancreatitis

57. 痔疮 hemorrhoids

58. 脾破裂 splenic rupture

59. 肝破裂 liver rupture

60. 阴道炎 vaginitis

61. 宫颈炎 cervicitis

62. 盆腔炎 pelvic infection

63. 月经失调 menstruation disorder

64. 功能性子宫出血 functional uterine bleeding

65. 妊娠（早孕）gestation（early pregnancy）

66. 宫外孕 ectopic/extrauterine pregnancy

67. 流产 miscarriage，abortion

68. 黄体破裂 rupture of corpus luteum

69. 荨麻疹 urticaria，hives

70. 湿疹 eczema

71. 接触性皮炎 contact dermatitis

72. 药物过敏 drug allergy

73. 过敏性紫癜 anaphylactoid purpura

74. 日光性皮炎 solar dermatitis

75. 痱子 heat rash

76. 单纯疱疹 herpes simplex virus

77. 带状疱疹 herpes zoster

78. 疣 verruca，wart

79. 结膜炎 conjunctivitis

80. 虹膜睫状体炎 iridocyclitis

81. 急性闭角型青光眼 acute angle-closure glaucoma

82. 结膜下出血 subconjunctival hemorrhage

83. 角膜炎 keratitis

84. 鼻炎 rhinitis，coryza

85. 急、慢性鼻窦炎 acute/chronic sinusitis/nasosinusitis

86. 急、慢性咽炎 acute/chronic pharyngitis

87. 急、慢性扁桃体炎 acute/chronic tonsillitis

88. 化脓性扁桃体炎 suppurative tonsillitis

89. 急、慢性喉炎 acute/chronic laryngitis

90. 喉头水肿 larynx edema

91. 声带小结 vocal nodules

92. 声带息肉 polyp of vocal cord

93. 耳廓外伤 auricle injuries

94. 鼓膜外伤 eardrum injuries

95. 鼓膜炎 myringitis

96. 中耳炎 tympanitis

97. 病毒性肝炎 viral hepatitis

98. 细菌性痢疾 bacillary dysentery

99. 伤寒 typhoid

100. 艾滋病 AIDS

101. 淋病 gonorrhea

102. 梅毒 syphilis

103. 麻疹 measles

104. 猩红热 scarlet fever

105. 流行性出血热 epidemic hemorrhagic fever

106. 流行性乙型脑炎 epidemic encephalitis B

107. 疟疾 malaria

108. 肺结核 tuberculosis

109. 流行性腮腺炎 mumps

110. 风疹 rubella

附录 B　医疗卫生机构名称

1. 医院 Hospital
2. 附属医院 Affiliated Hospital of … 或 Hospital Affiliated with/to …
3. 中心医院 Central Hospital
4. 专科医院 Specialized Hospital
5. 儿童医院 Children's Hospital
6. 中医医院 Traditional Chinese Medicine Hospital 或 TCM Hospital
7. 护理医院 Nursing Home 或 Nursing Hospital
8. 康复医院 Rehabilitation Hospital
9. 疗养院 Sanatorium 或 Convalescent Home 或 Convalescent Hospital
10. 胸科医院 Chest Hospital
11. 肺科医院 Lung Hospital
12. 妇产科医院；妇婴保健院 Women's Hospital 或 Maternity Hospital
13. 肝胆外科医院 Hepatobiliary Surgery Hospital
14. 精神卫生医院 Mental Health Hospital 或 Psychiatric Hospital
15. 脑科医院 Brain Hospital
16. 口腔医院 Stomatological Hospital 或 Oral Hospital
17. 眼耳鼻喉科医院 Eye and ENT Hospital
18. 眼科医院 Eye Hospital
19. 耳鼻喉科医院 ENT Hospital
20. 皮肤病医院 Dermatology Hospital
21. 性病医院 STD Hospital
22. 肛肠医院 Proctology Hospital
23. 肿瘤医院 Tumor Hospital 或 Oncology Hospital
24. 传染病防治院 Infectious Diseases Hospital
25. 口腔病防治院 Oral Clinic
26. 牙病防治院（所） Dental Clinic
27. 眼病防治院（所） Eye Clinic

28. 社区卫生服务中心 Community Healthcare Center

29. 社区卫生服务中心医疗服务站 Community Healthcare Clinic

30. 社区诊所 Community Clinic

31. 卫生室、医务室 Clinic 或 Medical Room

32. 公共卫生临床中心 Public Health Clinical Center

33. 疾病预防控制中心 Disease Control and Prevention Center

34. 医疗急救中心 Medical Emergency Center

35. 血液中心 Blood Center

36. 临床检验中心 Clinical Laboratory Center

37. 医保定点医疗机构 Medical Insurance Designated Hospital 或 Medical Insurance Designated Clinic

38. 医学科学技术情报研究所 Institute of Medical Science and Technology Information

39. 健康教育所 Health Education Center

40. 生物制品研究所 Research Institute of Biological Products

41. 肿瘤研究所 Oncology Institute

42. 气功研究所 *Qigong* Research Institute

43. 针灸经络研究所 Acupuncture and Meridian Research Institute

44. 免疫学研究所 Immunology Institute

45. 心血管研究所 Cardiovascular Medicine Institute

46. 放射医学研究所 Radiation Medicine Institute

47. 高血压研究所 Hypertension Research Institute

48. 伤骨科研究所 Orthopaedic Traumatology Institute

49. 内分泌研究所 Endocrinology Institute

50. 医保办 Medical Insurance Office

51. 血液管理办公室 Blood Management Office

52. 卫生监督所 Public Health Inspection Office

53. 红十字会 Red Cross Society

附录 C 医疗卫生服务类信息

1. 门诊部 Outpatient Department 或 Outpatients（用于 Department 可省略的场合）
2. 门诊楼 Outpatient Building 或 Outpatients（用于 Building 可省略的场合）
3. 急诊部 Emergency Department（Department 可以省略）
4. 急诊室 Emergency Clinic（Clinic 可以省略）
5. 急诊楼 Emergency Building（Building 可以省略）
6. 住院部 Inpatient Department
7. 病房、病区 Inpatient Ward
8. 病房楼 Inpatient Building
9. 医技楼 Medical Technology Building（Building 可以省略）
10. 检查室 Examination Room
11. 化验室 Laboratory 或 Lab
12. 治疗室 Treatment Room
13. 观察室 Observation Room
14. 候诊观察室 Waiting and Observation Room（Room 可以省略）
15. 抢救室 Emergency Room 或 Resuscitation Room（Room 均可以省略）
16. 现场抢救区 On-Site Emergency Care
17. 注射室 Injection Room
18. 输液室 Infusion Room
19. 注射输液室 Injection and Infusion Room
20. 配液室 Infusion Preparation Room
21. 手术室 Operating Room 或 Operating Theater
22. 麻醉室 Anesthesia Room
23. 苏醒室、恢复室 Recovery Room
24. 换药室 Dressing Room
25. 清创室 Wound Care Room 或 Debridement Room（Room 均可以省略）
26. 产房 Delivery Room

27. 重症监护室 Intensive Care Unit 或 ICU

28. 心脏重症监护室 Cardiac Care Unit 或 CCU

29. 冠心病重症监护室 Coronary Care Unit 或 CCU

30. 儿童重症监护室 Pediatric Intensive Care Unit 或 Pediatric ICU

31. 新生儿重症监护室 Neonatal Intensive Care Unit 或 NICU

32. 胎儿监护室 Fetus Monitoring Room（Room 可以省略）

33. 高压氧室、高压氧舱 Hyperbaric Oxygen Chamber

34. 预检处 Inquiries

35. 挂号处 Registration

36. 收费处 Cashier 或 Payment

37. 挂号、收费处 Registration and Payment

38. 自助挂号、自助挂号机 Self-Service Registration Machine（Machine 可以省略）

39. 住院手续办理处，住院登记处 Admission

40. 出院手续办理处 Discharge

41. 出入院办理处 Admission and Discharge

42. 处方 Prescription

43. 划价处、药品划价 Prescription Pricing

44. 取药处、医务室 Dispensary

45. 药房、西药房、中西药房 Pharmacy

46. 中药房 TCM Pharmacy

47. 中草药房 TCM Pharmacy（Herbal Medicine）

48. 中成药及西药房 Pharmacy（incl. Prepared Chinese Medicine）

49. 医保定点药店 Medical Insurance Designated Pharmacy

50. 用药咨询处 Medication Consultation

51. 门诊煎药处 Outpatient Herbal Medicine Decoction Service

52. 叫号台 Calling Desk

53. 候诊区 Waiting Area

54. 就诊区 Outpatient Area

55. 诊室 Consulting Room

56. 第……诊室 Consulting Room ...

57. 男诊室 Men's Consulting Room

58. 女诊室 Women's Consulting Room

59. 乙肝病毒携带者诊室 HBV Carriers' Consulting Room

60. 登记处 Registry

61. 预约处 Appointments

62. 自助预约机 Self-Service Appointment Machine（Machine 可以省略）

63. 检查、化验等候区 Lab Test Waiting Area

64. 取报告处 Lab Report Collection

65. 取检查、化验结果处 Lab Test Reports

66. 标本登记处 Specimen Registration

67. 标本接收处 Specimen Collection

68. 放标本处 Specimens

69. 抽血处 Blood Sampling

70. 静脉采血处 Venous Blood Sampling Room

71. 普通取血处 Routine Blood Sampling Room

72. 隔离取血处 Isolated Blood Sampling Room

73. 拍片室、摄片室 Radiography Room

74. 暗室 Darkroom

75. 冲片室 Film Developing Room

76. 读片室、阅片室 Film Reading Room

77. 护士站 Nurses Station

78. 医生办公室 Doctor's Office

79. 配餐室 Meal Preparation Room（Room 可以省略）

80. 营养室 Nutrition Room

81. 宣教室 Health Education Room（Room 可以省略）

82. 盥洗室 Wash Area

83. 院内小卖部 Store

84. 亲友等候区 Visitors Waiting Area

85. 会客区 Reception Area

86. 血液中心 Blood Center

87. 血库 Blood Bank

88. 血液采集区 Blood Collection Area

89. 献血前等候区 Donors Waiting Lounge

90. 献血前检测区 Donors Blood Test Area

91. 献血咨询登记处 Donation Counseling and Registration

92. 献血后休息区 Donors Rest Lounge

93. 医用电梯 Medical Service Elevator 或 Medical Use Only（用于 Elevator 可省略场合）

94. 手术室专用电梯 Operating Room Elevator 或 Operating Room Only（用于 Elevator 可省略

场合）

95. 医疗急救电话 120 First Aid Call 120

96. 救护车 Ambulance

97. 隔离区 Isolation Area 或 Quarantine Area

98. 清洁区 Sterile Area 或 Cleanroom

99. 半污染区 Buffer Area

100. 污染区 Contaminated Area

101. 污物间 Soiled Articles Disposal Room（Room 可以省略）

102. 生活垃圾（存放处）（指非医用垃圾）Non-Medical Waste

103. 医用垃圾（存放处）（指医用废弃物等）Medical Waste

104. 消毒产品检验受理处 Sterile Items Test Registration

105. 急诊办公室 Emergency Department Office

106. 门诊办公室 Outpatient Department Office

107. 门诊接待室 Reception Room（Room 可以省略）

108. 医护部 Medical and Nursing Department

109. 护理部 Nursing Department

110. 投诉电话、投诉热线 Complaints Hotline

111. 投诉与建议箱 Complaints and Suggestions

112. 医疗纠纷处理办公室 Complaints Office

113. 预防保健科 Preventive Medicine Department

114. 院感科 Hospital-Acquired Infection Control Department

115. 太平间、停尸房 Mortuary 或 Morgue

116. 亲友告别室 Visitation Room

117. 当心射线 CAUTION! Radiation

118. 锐器！请注意 CAUTION! Sharp Objects

119. 易燃物品 Flammable Materials

120. 剧毒物品 Toxic Materials

121. 生物危险，请勿入内 DANGER! Biohazard! No Admittance

122. 患者止步 Staff Only

123. 请勿谈论病人隐私 Please Respect the Privacy of Our Patients

124. 男宾止步 Women Only

125. 请在诊室外候诊 Please Wait Outside the Consulting Room

126. 医疗急救通道 Emergency Access

127. 进入实验区，请穿好工作服 Lab Area//Lab Coats Required

128. 血液告急 Urgent! Blood Donors Needed Now!

129. 血液告急，请伸出您的手臂！ Donate blood，help save lives!

130. 专家门诊 Expert Clinic

131. 特需门诊 Special Need Clinic

132. 特约门诊 Special Appointment Clinic

133. 预约门诊 Advance Appointment Clinic

134. 隔离门诊 Isolation Clinic

135. 中医门诊 Traditional Chinese Medicine Clinic/或 TCM Clinic

136. 护理门诊 Nursing Clinic

137. 专科门诊 Specialist Clinic

138. 发热门诊 Fever Clinic

139. 腹泻门诊 Diarrhea Clinic

140. 营养门诊 Nutrition Clinic

141. 镇痛门诊 Aches and Pains Clinic

142. 肥胖症门诊 Obesity Clinic

143. 职业病咨询门诊 Occupational Health Consulting Clinic

144. 门诊须知 Outpatient Guide

145. 急诊须知 Emergency Patient Guide

146. 病员须知 Patient Guide

147. 住院须知 Admission Guide

148. 取报告须知 Lab Report Collection Guide

149. 患者入口 Patients Entrance

150. 探视入口 Visitors Entrance

151. 探视时间 Visiting Hours

152. 探视须知 Visitors' Guide

153. 心理咨询 Psychological Counseling

154. 免疫预防接种 Vaccination and Immunization

155. 更年期保健 Menopause Health Care

156. 危机干预 Crisis Intervention

157. 医学美容 Medical Cosmetology Department 或 Medical Cosmetology

158. 营养咨询 Nutrition Counseling

159. 献血体检 Blood Donor Health Check

160. 健康体检、常规体检 Health Checkup 或 Physical Examination

161. 口腔修复 Prosthodontics

162. 口腔预防 Preventive Dentistry

163. 口腔正畸 Orthodontics Clinic

164. 口腔种植 Oral Implantology

165. 人工牙齿种植 Dental Implantology

166. 远程会诊 Teleconsulation

167. 远程医疗 Telemedicine

168. 生物安全 Bio-safety

169. 无偿献血 Voluntary Blood Donation

附录 D 医疗科室名称

1. 病理科 Pathology Department（Department 可以省略）

2. 产科 Obstetrics Department（Department 可以省略）

3. 超声科 Ultrasonography Lab（Lab 可以省略）

4. 传染科 Infectious Diseases Department

5. 儿科 Pediatric Department（Department 可以省略）

6. 儿内科 Pediatric Internal Medicine Department（Department 可以省略）

7. 儿外科 Pediatric Surgery Department（Department 可以省略）

8. 耳鼻（咽）喉科 Otolaryngology Department 或 Ear, Nose and Throat Department 或 E. N. T. Department（Department 可以省略）

9. 放射介入科 Radioactive Intervention Department（Department 可以省略）

10. 放射科 Radiology Department（Department 可以省略）

11. 风湿科 Rheumatology Department（Department 可以省略）

12. 风湿免疫科 Rheumatology and Immunology Department（Department 可以省略）

13. 妇科 Gynecology Department（Department 可以省略）

14. 妇女保健科 Women's Health Care Department（Department 可以省略）

15. 腹腔镜外科 Laparoscope Surgery Department（Department 可以省略）

16. 肝胆科 Hepatology Department（Department 可以省略）

17. 肝胆外科 Hepatological Surgery Department（Department 可以省略）

18. 肝炎科 Hepatitis Department

19. 肛肠科 Proctology Department

20. 痔科 Hemorrhoid Department

21. 高血压科 Hypertension Department

22. 骨科、骨伤科 Orthopedics Department（Department 可以省略）

23. 核医学科 Nuclear Medicine Department（Department 可以省略）

24. 呼吸内科 Respiratory Medicine Department（Department 可以省略）

25. 检验科 Clinical Lab

26. 介入科 Intervention Department

27. 戒毒科 Drug Rehabilitation Department（Department 可以省略）或 Drug Rehab Department（Department 可以省略）

28. 精神科 Psychiatry Department

29. 康复科 Rehabilitation Department（Department 可以省略）或 Rehabilitation Medicine Department（Department 可以省略）

30. 康复医学科 Rehabilitation Medicine Department（Department 可以省略）

31. 口腔科 Stomatology Department（Department 可以省略）

32. 口腔外科 Oral Surgery Department（Department 可以省略）

33. 老年病科 Geriatric Department 或 Geriatrics（用于 Department 可以省略的场合）

34. 麻醉科 Anesthesiology Department（Department 可以省略）

35. 泌尿科 Urology Department（Department 可以省略）

36. 免疫科 Immunology Department（Department 可以省略）

37. 男科、男性科 Andrology Department（Department 可以省略）

38. 内分泌科 Endocrinology Department（Department 可以省略）

39. 内科 Internal Medicine Department（Department 可以省略）

40. 皮肤科 Dermatology Department（Department 可以省略）

41. 普通内科、通用内科 General Internal Medicine Department（Department 可以省略）

42. 普通外科 General Surgery Department（Department 可以省略）

43. 器官移植科 Organ Transplantation Department（Department 可以省略）

44. 伤科 Traumatology Department（Department 可以省略）

45. 烧伤科 Burns Department

46. 神经内科 Neurology Department（Department 可以省略）

47. 神经外科 Neurosurgery Department（Department 可以省略）

48. 肾内科 Nephrology Department（Department 可以省略）

49. 生殖健康科 Reproductive Health Care Department（Department 可以省略）

50. 生殖科 Reproductive Medicine Department（Department 可以省略）

51. 手外科 Hand Surgery Department（Department 可以省略）

52. 输血科 Blood Transfusion Department（Department 可以省略）

53. 体验中心 Physical Examination Center/Health Checkup Center

54. 外科 Surgery Department（Department 可以省略）

55. 微创外科 Minimally Invasive Surgery Department（Department 可以省略）

56. 消化内科 Gastroenterology Department（Department 可以省略）或 Gastrology Department（Department 可以省略）

57. 心理科 Psychology Department（Department 可以省略）

58. 心理咨询科 Psychology Counseling Department（Department 可以省略）

59. 心外科 Cardiac Surgery Department（Department 可以省略）

60. 心胸外科 Cardiothoracic Surgery Department（Department 可以省略）

61. 心血管内科 Cardiovascular Medicine Department（Department 可以省略）

62. 心脏介入科 Cardiovascular Intervention Department（Department 可以省略）

63. 心胸科 Cardiology Department（Department 可以省略）

64. 新生儿外科 Neonatal Surgery Department（Department 可以省略）

65. 新生儿医疗中心 Neonatal Medicine Center

66. 性病科 Sexually Transmitted Diseases Department 或 STD Department

67. 胸外科 Thoracic Surgery Department（Department 可以省略）

68. 血管介入科 Vascular Intervention Department（Department 可以省略）

69. 血管外科 Vascular Surgery Department（Department 可以省略）

70. 血液科 Hematology Department（Department 可以省略）

71. 牙科 Dental Department 或 Dentistry

72. 眼科 Ophthalmology Department（Department 可以省略）

73. 医学心理科 Medical Psychology Department（Department 可以省略）

74. 针灸科 Acupuncture Department（Department 可以省略）

75. 整形外科 Plastic Surgery Department（Department 可以省略）

76. 正颌正畸科 Maxillofacial Surgery and Orthodontics Department（Department 可以省略）

77. 中医科 Traditional Chinese Medicine Department（Department 可以省略）或 TCM Department（Department 可以省略）

78. 中医儿科 TCM Pediatrics Department（Department 可以省略）

79. 中医妇科 TCM Gynecology Department（Department 可以省略）

80. 中医骨病治疗科 TCM Orthopedics Department（Department 可以省略）

81. 中医理疗科 TCM Physiotherapy Department（Department 可以省略）

82. 肿瘤科 Oncology Department（Department 可以省略）

83. 综合治疗科 Integrated Therapy Department（Department 可以省略）

附录 E 其他医学专有名词

• 检查化验项目

1. 体温测量 temperature taking
2. 量血压 blood pressure measurement
3. 动态血压检查 ambulatory blood pressure monitoring(可以缩写为 ABPM)
4. 功能检查 function test
5. 白带检查 leucorrhea examination
6. 肺功能检查 pulmonary function test
7. 眼科验光 optometry
8. 免疫检查 immunoassay
9. 智力测量 intelligence assessment
10. 心理测验 psychological test
11. 妊高症监测 gestational hypertension monitoring
12. 常规化验 routine test
13. 儿保化验 child care test
14. 尿液化验 urine test
15. 粪便化验 excrement test
16. 妇科化验 gynecological test
17. 宫颈冷冻 cervical cryotherapy
18. 白带化验 leucorrhea test
19. 血气分析 arterial blood gas analysis
20. B 超 B-mode ultrasound
21. 阴超 transvaginal ultrasound
22. 彩超 color ultrasound
23. 腹部 B 超 abdominal ultrasound scan
24. 心脏超声波 cardiac ultrasound scan 或 echocardiography

25. X 光摄片 X-ray radiography
26. 断层扫描(CT) CT scan
27. 断层扫描(发射单光子计算机) ECT 或 Emission computed tomography
28. 透视 fluoroscopy 或 X-ray
29. 核磁共振 MRI 或 magnetic resonance imaging
30. 口腔放射 oral radiology
31. 牙片 dental film
32. 数字牙片 digital dental film
33. 乳腺摄片 galactophore radiography 或 mammogram
34. 心电图 ECG
35. 动态心电图 DCG 或 dynamic electrocardiogram 或 holter monitor
36. 脑、肌电图 electroencephalography and electromyography 或 EEG and EMG
37. 胃肠电图 electrogastrogram 或 EGG
38. 内窥镜检查 endoscopy
39. 胃镜检查 gastroscopy
40. 肠镜检查 enteroscopy
41. 支气管镜检查 bronchoscopy
42. 胃十二指肠镜检查 gastroduodenoscopy
43. 艾滋病初筛实验 HIV Screening 或 HIV/AIDS Screening
44. 骨密度检测 bone mineral density test
45. 听力测试 audiometry
46. 红外线扫描 infrared ray
47. 快速检测 rapid test

• 医疗措施

48. 理疗 physical therapy 或 physiotherapy
49. 放疗 radiation oncology 或 radiotherapy
50. 弱视治疗 amblyopia treatment
51. 中医科按摩 TCM(massage therapy)
52. 推拿 tuina 或 manipulation
53. 针灸 acupuncture
54. 预防接种 prophylactic vaccination
55. 新生儿水疗抚触 neonatal hydrotherapy and massage
56. 心导管术 cardiac catheterization

57. 心理治疗 psychotherapy

58. 骨髓移植 bone marrow transplantation

59. 透析 dialysis

60. 血透 hemodialysis

61. 钴 60 治疗；同位素治疗 cobalt-60 treatment 或 isotope treatment

62. 助听器验配 hearing aid fitting

63. 高压氧治疗 hyperbaric oxygen therapy

64. 功能训练 functional training

• 医学保障设置

65. 病案室；病史室 Medical Records Room（Room 可以省略）

66. 疫苗室 Vaccination Room（Room 可以省略）

67. 药械科 Drug and Equipment Department（Department 可以省略）

68. 操作室 Procedure Room

69. 放射防护 Radiation Protection

70. 放射物品 Radioactive Materials

71. 供应保障组 Supply Team

72. 供应室 Storage and Supply Room

73. 供应保障区 Storage and Supply Area

74. 实验区 Laboratory Area

75. 实验室 Laboratory 或 Lab

76. 生化实验室 Biochemistry Lab

77. 病毒实验室 Virus Analysis Lab

78. 毒理实验室 Toxicology Lab

79. 免疫实验室 Immunoassay Lab

80. 放射免疫实验室 Radioimmunoassay Lab 或 RIA Lab

81. 分子生物学实验室 Molecular Biology Lab

82. 微量元素实验室 Trace Element Lab

83. 微生物实验室 Microbiology Lab

84. 细胞化验室 Cell Lab

85. 细菌培养室 Bacterial Culture Lab

86. 细菌室 Bacteriology Lab

87. 血液实验室 Blood Analysis Lab

参考书目

[1] Bickley，L. S. *Bates' Guide to Physical Examination and History Taking*[M]. 12th edition. Philadelphia：Williams & Wilkins，2013.

[2] Swartz，M. H. *Textbook of Physical Diagnosis：History and Examination*[M]. 7th edition. Philadelphia：Elsevier Saunders，2014.

[3] Adam，L.C.，肖幸锐.实用医学英语会话——医生篇[M].北京：中国水利水电出版社，2007.

[4] Adam，L.C.，肖幸锐.实用医学英语会话——护士篇[M].北京：中国水利水电出版社，2008.

[5] Gyorff，M.医生诊疗英语会话[M].上海：复旦大学出版社，2013.

[6] Glendinning，E. H.，& R. Howard.剑桥医学英语[M].北京：人民邮电出版社，2010.

[7] 北京市教育委员会.北京奥运会英语口语读本[M].初级本，高级本.北京：北京师范大学出版社，2008.

[8] 顾民，武晓泓.门诊常用医学会话[M].南京：江苏凤凰科学技术出版社，2018.

[9] 刘虹，乔玉玲.医学英语会话[M].北京：北京大学医学出版社，2009.

[10] 唐熠达，冉志华.住院医师英语手册[M].北京：人民卫生出版社，2015.

[11] 魏葆霖.大学英语口语套路词典[M].上海：华东师范大学出版社，2003.

[12] 王文秀，李志红，冯永平.医务英语会话[M].北京：人民卫生出版社，2001.

[13] 王文秀，王颖，贾轶群.临床医师实用英语[M].2 版.北京：人民卫生出版社，2009.

[14] 中国国家标准化管理委员会.GB/T 30240.1—2013 公共服务领域英文译写规范第 7 部分：医疗卫生[S].北京：中国标准出版社，2017.

[15] 曾广翘.医生诊疗英语会话[M].上海：复旦大学出版社，2005.

[16] 赵贵旺，粟为农.医学英语视听说[M].青岛：中国海洋大学出版社，2008.

[17] Ciolli，C. Beyond the Handshake：How People Greet Each Other Around the World.（2020 - 04 - 09）[2020 - 05 - 24]. http://www. afar. com/magazine/beyond-the-handshake-how-people-greet-each-other-around-the-world.

[18] Debby，M. Polite Words and Phrases.（2020 - 03 - 16）[2020 - 04 - 20]. https://www. thespruce. com/polite-words-and-phrases - 1216714.

[19] Fraley，L. What to Know About COVID-19 Diagnosis.（2020 - 03 - 05）[2020 - 05 - 24]. http://www. healthline. com/health/coronavirus-diagnosis.

[20] Khatri，M. What Is My Medical History.（2018 - 09 - 18）[2020 - 03 - 02]. http://www. webmd. com/a-to-z-guides/what-is-my-medical-history#1.